Healthy, Wealthy, and Wise

*The Hoover Institution gratefully acknowledges
the following individuals and foundations
for their significant support of this publication:*

JAN AND JIM BOCHNOWSKI
LYNDE AND HARRY BRADLEY FOUNDATION
FOUNDATION FOR BETTER HEALTH

Healthy, Wealthy, and Wise

5 Steps to a Better Health Care System

SECOND EDITION

John F. Cogan,
R. Glenn Hubbard, and
Daniel P. Kessler

THE HOOVER INSTITUTION PRESS

Stanford University ▪ *Stanford, California*

and

THE AEI PRESS

Publisher for the American Enterprise Institute ▪ *Washington, D.C.*

THE HOOVER INSTITUTION ON WAR, REVOLUTION AND PEACE, *founded at Stanford University in 1919 by Herbert Hoover, who went on to become the thirty-first president of the United States, is an interdisciplinary research center for advanced study on domestic and international affairs.*

www.hoover.org

AEI THE AMERICAN ENTERPRISE INSTITUTE *is a community of scholars and supporters committed to expanding liberty, increasing individual opportunity, and strengthening free enterprise.*

www.aei.org

Hoover Institution Press Publication No. 582

Hoover Institution at Leland Stanford Junior University,
Stanford, California 94305-6010

First edition 2005
Second edition, first printing 2011

17 16 15 14 13 12 11   7 6 5 4 3 2 1

Manufactured in the United States of America
The paper used in this publication meets the minimum Requirements of the American National Standard for Information Sciences—Permanence of Paper for Printed Library Materials, ANSI/NISO Z39.48-1992. ∞

Cataloging-in-Publication Data is available from the Library of Congress.
ISBN-13: 978-0-8179-1064-8 (cloth. : alk. paper)
ISBN-13: 978-0-8179-1066-2 (e-book)

Contents

Preface to the Second Edition

When we published the first edition of this book in 2005, our country faced an important fork in the road in health policy: shift to more patient-centered health care, with incentives to control costs and promote innovation, or surrender to pressure for expansion of the role of government, with diminished incentives for both cost containment and innovation. With the passage of the Patient Protection and Affordable Care Act (PPACA) in 2010, President Obama and the Congress chose the second path.

This new law represents a wrong turn. Unpopular with the American people in no small part because of the uncompromising legislative process through which it was enacted, the law put the crucial first step of cost containment and innovation in the back seat of a car driven by costly expansion of access within a system of flawed incentives. This approach will lead to higher health spending, greater government involvement in health care administration, and negative effects on the U.S. economic activity.

There is a better way.

Fundamental reform centering on tax changes, insurance-market changes, and the redesign of Medicare and Medicaid can slow the rate of growth of health care costs, expand access to high-quality health care, and slow down the runaway budget train. While we wish the PPACA had not been passed and we believe Congress should start over, we also present pathways toward sensible reform within the recently enacted law and, importantly, within the existing frameworks of the Medicare and Medicaid programs.

It remains the case that unintended consequences of a handful of public policies are in large part responsible for the problems of the health care system. These policies share a common feature, now amplified by the PPACA: they fail to promote the proper functioning of markets. In two areas in particular, tax policy and health insurance regulation, government policy continues to actively hinder the operation of markets for health services.

Since the book's initial publication, we have conducted additional research on the consequences of tax policy for health spending and health insurance. We present that work, along with updated estimates of the impact of our proposal on the federal budget, the number of insured Americans, and health care spending.

Our closing point in the first edition is now more true after the passage of the 2010 law: the time to implement sensible reforms is *now*. Failure to do so will exacerbate the problems of wasteful cost growth and lack of insurance. It will inevitably increase the pressure for more public intervention, with adverse consequences for the quality of health care and economic growth more broadly.

John F. Cogan   *R. Glenn Hubbard*   *Daniel P. Kessler*

Acknowledgments

We are grateful to Joe Antos, Chris DeMuth, Doug Holtz-Eakin, Al Hubbard, Ben Lytle, Cindy Miller, Sam Nussbaum, Mark Pauly, Dhan Shapurji, Marc Sumerlin, and Janet Stokes Trantwein for helpful comments and discussions; to Evan Lodes for exceptional research assistance; and to Sam Thernstrom and Barbara Egbert for excellent editorial advice.

Introduction

Health care in the United States has made remarkable advances over the past forty years. Dramatic improvements in medical technology have expanded both the length and quality of life. In general, Americans are remarkably satisfied with the quality of their health care. Yet our health care system also has several well-known problems: high costs, significant numbers of people without insurance, and glaring gaps in quality and efficiency.

How can we preserve the strengths of this system while addressing its weaknesses? Policymakers, like Americans as a whole, are divided about whether health reform should focus on increasing the role of individuals or of government. Supporters of individual choice and markets point out that these mechanisms provide consumer satisfaction in most situations; health care should be no different. Supporters of increased public intervention argue that our health care system's problems prove that individual involvement has failed. According to this reasoning, imperfect information, irrationality, and insufficient competition should give government a more prominent role.

In our view, the argument for increased public intervention is seriously flawed. As we discuss in the following chapters, the unintended consequences of a handful of longstanding public policies are in large part responsible for the problems of the health care system. These policies share a common feature: they fail to promote cost-conscious behavior and competition. Such incentives permeate both private markets and government programs like Medicare and Medicaid. The central goal of health reform must be to change these flawed policies.

Most importantly, tax policy and insurance regulation have actively hindered the operation of private markets for health services. The recently enacted Patient Protection and Affordable Care Act (PPACA) of 2010, by failing to address these issues and by adding another layer of misguided regulations, will only make matters worse. Current tax policy generally allows people to deduct employer-provided health-insurance expenditures, but requires direct out-of-pocket medical spending to come from after-tax income. This tax preference has given consumers the incentive to purchase health care through low-deductible, low-copayment insurance instead of paying for it out-of-pocket. This type of insurance has led to today's U.S. health care market, in which cost-unconsciousness and wasteful medical practices are the norm. Insurance regulation, by requiring health plans to cover certain types of care and restricting their ability to set premiums, has raised insurance costs and limited the available range of insurance options. These inefficiencies have been an important factor contributing to the rising number of uninsured people.

Poor design of government programs has similarly discouraged cost-consciousness. This flaw has, in turn, led to unsustainable cost growth. Medicare's low copayments have left beneficiaries with little responsibility for the cost of their care—or "skin in the game"—thereby attenuating incentives to limit their use of services. Although Medicaid's low copayments are understandable, the current structure of the program allows both federal and state governments to avoid bearing budgetary responsibility for their benefits and eligibility decisions and thereby creates powerful disincentives for cost control.

In three other areas—the provision of health care information, the enforcement of antitrust laws, and the creation of medical malpractice rules—government policy has failed to give individuals and health care providers the tools to make sensible choices.

As a general rule, markets work well when information about product and service prices and quality is widely available. Although recently the federal government has taken steps to disseminate information about health care prices and quality to both consumers and providers, much more needs to be done to ensure that health care markets perform their essential role of promoting lower cost and higher quality.

Markets also work well when vigorous competition among suppliers prevails. Government enforcement of antitrust laws in health care markets has been too lax. As a consequence, health care providers are able to engage in anticompetitive practices that drive up prices and reduce quality.

Finally, markets work well when appropriate penalties are levied on suppliers of deficient products and negligent service providers. Current medical malpractice law imposes excessive penalties that have led to costly defensive practices and higher rates of medical errors.

The first steps in solving the problems of the U.S. health system must include changing these policies.

In this book, we propose five reforms to improve the ability of markets to create a lower-cost, higher-quality health care system that is responsive to the needs of individuals. These reforms are summarized in box 1:

1. **Increase individual involvement.** For the private health care market, we propose three changes to the tax code, designed to reduce the distorting role of third-party payers, encourage saving for future health care needs, and reduce the rate of uninsurance. For government health programs, we propose to shift beneficiaries' financial responsibility toward higher copayments and away from premiums.

2. **Deregulate insurance markets and redesign Medicare and Medicaid.** We propose allowing insurance companies to offer health plans on a nationwide basis, free from costly state benefit mandates and excessive rate regulation, to foster more portable, more affordable health insurance. We also propose a subsidy for persistently high-cost individuals. We propose repeal of the 2010 PPACA's insurance mandates, subsidies,

and misguided regulations. For Medicare, we propose expanding the role of private health plans in the delivery of health care benefits; for Medicaid, we propose to block-grant federal support to the states.

3. **Improve provision of information.** We propose public–private partnerships to provide better information to doctors and patients.

4. **Enhance competition.** We propose greater federal scrutiny of anticompetitive behavior by hospitals and other health care providers and stricter application of antitrust laws when such behavior is found.

5. **Reform the malpractice system.** We propose malpractice reform to reduce wasteful treatment and medical errors.

We also propose further study of a sixth reform: revocation or limitation of the current tax preference for nonprofits.

In combination, these reforms will reduce health care costs by approximately $84 billion per year without reducing the quality of care. These savings will accrue to consumers and workers. Decreases in health spending will lead to decreases in health-insurance costs. And just as increases in health-insurance costs are borne by workers in the form of lower wages, decreases will accrue to them as higher wages.

Cost savings, however, are only one of our goals; our policies will also improve the system's productivity, fairness, and responsiveness. For example, improved health information and malpractice reform will improve quality. Tax reform will make the tax treatment of health expenses more progressive, with the largest gains for low-income households.

BOX 1
Proposed Reforms

1. Increase individual involvement
   - Make all health care expenses tax deductible
   - Expand health savings accounts
   - Provide tax credits for low-income individuals and families
   - Increase copayments in government insurance programs

2. Deregulate insurance markets and redesign Medicare and Medicaid
   - Create a federal market for insurance for individuals and small groups similar to that already enjoyed by large employers that self-insure
   - Subsidize private insurance for the chronically ill
   - Repeal recently enacted mandates and some insurance regulations
   - Expand role of private sector health plans in Medicare
   - Block-grant federal support for Medicaid

3. Improve provision of information
   - Expand the number and scope of report cards on doctors and hospitals
   - Promote use of "best practices" through guidelines

4. Enhance competition

5. Reform the malpractice system

Reducing wasteful spending and inefficient regulation will reduce uninsurance. We estimate that our reforms will provide insurance to at least 7 million—and perhaps as many as 21 million—currently uninsured people. (The wide range of that estimate reflects the considerable uncertainty about the effects of various policies on the uninsured.)

These reforms will also gradually but fundamentally give individuals more control over and choices for their health care. Most notably, tax deductibility and health savings accounts reduce the financial penalty for purchasing medical care directly rather than through employer-provided insurance. Consumers will respond by shifting the type of insurance they purchase to lower-cost catastrophic insurance and away from first-dollar coverage. As the availability of health care report cards and other user-friendly information devices increases, consumers will become better equipped to make health care decisions, and as consumers spend less on insurance premiums and more on direct medical-care purchases, health care providers will become more responsive to their demands than to those of insurance bureaucracies.

Nationwide insurance with fewer mandates will expand the number of insurance choices available. In conjunction with more vigorous enforcement of antitrust laws against health care providers, this enhanced competition in insurance markets will reduce the cost of insurance for everyone, but likely most for non-group markets in rural areas where coverage options are currently narrow. Tax credits, by providing additional health care resources to persons with low and moderate incomes, will make health insurance more financially attractive and broaden insurance options. As coverage increases and more relatively healthy individuals join health-insurance pools, the range of options will continue to expand and the cost will decline further.

At the same time, our policies will not abruptly alter the existing system of employer-sponsored health insurance. As we describe below, the tax reforms we propose retain significant incentives for employers to provide health insurance. Our proposed reforms benefit the individual and the employer market alike. We are agnostic about the ultimate balance that should be struck between individual and employer-based insurance; to the extent that they are efficiently able to pool together persons with different health care risks, employers should continue to provide insurance. However, we firmly believe that this balance should be determined by market forces seeking to deliver the care that individuals want—at the cost they are willing to pay.

Our book proceeds in three chapters. In chapter 1, we outline the challenge facing public policy: retaining and continuing to achieve gains to society from the U.S. health care system while minimizing its costs, both financial and otherwise. Chapter 2 proposes a market-based approach to accomplishing this goal, explaining why the most important problems with our health care system are in large part due to five flawed public policies, and showing how five sets of specific reforms can correct these flaws. Chapter 3 quantifies the expected consequences of our reforms, based on estimates of how consumers and providers have responded to past changes in markets for health care, and explains how we calculate their effects on health spending, the uninsured, and the federal budget.

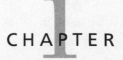

CHAPTER 1

The Challenge: Obtaining High-Quality, Affordable Health Care

Everyone agrees that, over the past fifty years, the U.S. health care system has yielded vast benefits for large numbers of Americans. Yet there are many instances in which today's health care is costly and wasteful, leaving people without appropriate care. The challenge for public policy is to find a way to keep the (good) sophisticated health care procedures in instances where they are productive, but avoid the (bad) wasteful spending and uninsurance.

The Good: Innovation

Evidence of the U.S. health care system's innovative strength is overwhelming. In the 1940s, the discovery of a low-cost process for manufacturing penicillin contributed significantly to the triumph of modern medicine over infectious disease.[1] The Nobel prizes in medicine and physiology have been awarded to more Americans than to researchers in all other countries combined. Eight of the ten most important medical innovations of the past thirty years originated in the United States.[2] Eight of the world's ten top-selling drugs are produced by companies headquartered in the United States.[3]

American consumers recognize the benefits of this system. Survey evidence on this point is clear: 82 percent of Americans are satisfied with the quality of health care they receive; 86 percent are satisfied with their doctors and nurses; and 74 percent rate the quality of hospitals in their area as good or excellent.[4]

The remarkable success we have had in treating cardiovascular disease is a good demonstration of the strengths of our health care system.[5] Beginning in the 1960s, mortality from cardiovascular disease in the United States began to decline rapidly, falling about 2 percent each year from 1960 to 1995; the cumulative decline over this period was close to two-thirds. To put this dramatic change into context, the decline in mortality from cardiovascular disease explains essentially all of the overall reduction in mortality for the elderly since 1965. For the population as a whole, 98 percent of the reduction in mortality was a result of our progress in fighting cardiovascular disease. There are several causes for this decline in cardiovascular mortality, but evidence indicates that medical care (rather than changes in health behaviors, such as smoking) accounts for a relatively large share of it.[6]

The medical care behind this revolution in cardiovascular health is strongly related to the incentives for innovation in the U.S. system. According to a 2002 study that analyzed the findings of research teams from seventeen countries, the United States has been one of the leading countries—if not the leading country—in promoting the use of intensive medical treatment for serious cardiac disease (see box 2).[7] Generous payments for treatment for heart attack in America led to the early adoption and widespread use of technologically advanced treatments. Countries with weaker incentives for the adoption and implementation of costly technology use these procedures much less.

Were the introduction and diffusion of these costly intensive cardiac procedures in the United States beneficial? On the whole, cost-benefit calculations suggest they were.[8]

The typical forty-five-year-old American can expect to have $30,000 spent on his behalf to treat cardiovascular disease over his remaining lifetime. These treatments can be expected to extend this person's life by approximately three years, worth (in economic terms) approximately $120,000. On average, each dollar spent on cardiovascular care generates four dollars' worth of benefits.[9]

New drugs for depression offer another example of the benefits of innovation. Eli Lilly's introduction of Prozac in 1988, followed by the development of several related compounds, revolutionized treatment of this common and debilitating mental illness. These new pharmaceuticals are as effective as their predecessors, are safer and easier to administer, and have fewer adverse side effects, making them more attractive to both physicians and patients. They are also, however, substantially more expensive than their older, off-patent counterparts. Despite their high cost, the

BOX 2
The Use of Cardiac Procedures in Nine Countries

Countries differ widely in their incentives for, and use of, advanced technological procedures to treat cardiac illness. Some provide weak incentives for adoption and use of technology, including global hospital budgets, salaried compensation of physicians, and limits on capital equipment purchases. Others provide strong incentives, including generous payments to physicians and hospitals for the provision of additional intensive treatment. Countries also differ in how extensively they use advanced cardiac procedures. For instance, the gold-standard, high-tech diagnostic procedure used to assess artery status is cardiac catheterization or angiography, which may be followed

(continued on facing page)

FIGURE 1
The Relationship between Incentives and the Use of Intensive Cardiac Procedures

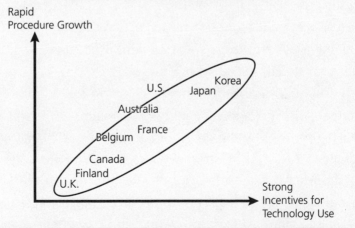

Source: Mark McClellan and Daniel Kessler, eds., *A Global Analysis of Technological Change in Health Care: Heart Attack* (Ann Arbor. University of Michigan Press, 2002).

(Box 2 *continued*)

by either coronary artery bypass graft surgery or percutaneous transluminal coronary angioplasty to "revascularize," or remove, arterial blockages.

Figure 1 summarizes the relationship, reported by Mark McClellan and Daniel Kessler, between incentives for the use of these three procedures in 1995 and the growth in their use from 1991 to 1995.[10] As figure 1 shows, there is a strong relationship between incentives and procedure growth. Japan and Korea have the strongest incentives for intensive cardiac procedures and the fastest rate of growth. Although pure fee-for-service reimbursement of health care expenses is rarer in the United States and Australia, significant private financing for health services and a lack of formal constraints on hospitals' use of new technologies have led to very rapid growth in procedure use in those countries as well. France, Belgium, and some Canadian provinces have intermediate incentives and intermediate growth rates; Finland, the United Kingdom, and other Canadian provinces have more limited incentives and the slowest growth in procedure use.

discovery and diffusion of these new pharmaceuticals have been another good health care investment, with every dollar spent on them returning six to seven dollars in societal benefits.[11]

These two examples illustrate the potential importance to public policy of preserving incentives for innovation in the U.S. system. At least for cardiac and mental health care, no one would like to turn back the medical-care clock to the 1950s, even if it meant that they could spend the money they saved on something else.

The Bad: High Costs and a
Large Uninsured Population

While Americans generally approve of the quality of their health care, they have two main concerns with it: high costs and the number of individuals without insurance.

HIGH COSTS: NO EASY ANSWER

In 2008, the United States spent $7,538 per capita on medical care, or 16 percent of its gross domestic product (GDP), compared to $4,079 in Canada (10.4 percent of GDP), $3,737 in Germany (10.5 percent), and $3,129 in the United Kingdom (8.7 percent).[12] Premiums for employer-sponsored health plans doubled from 2000 to 2009.[13] Although Americans are generally pleased with the quality of care they receive, surveys show that they are not happy with its cost. In 2010, 82 percent rated the quality of their care to be "good" or "excellent," but 76 percent reported feeling dissatisfied with the cost.[14]

However, spending a large share of GDP on medical care is not necessarily bad.[15] If the spending is "worth it"—if it improves the health of patients enough to justify the cost— then rising health spending should be of no greater concern than the increasing spending on, for example, information technology. The problem is that a lot of U.S. health care spending provides few or no measurable health benefits for the individuals who receive the care. In many cases, diagnostic procedures and tests are over-utilized, procedures are employed without tangible results, and expensive pharmaceuticals are unnecessarily prescribed.

Unfortunately, productive care and wasteful care are not so easy to tell apart. Even care that provides well-recognized benefits to the vast majority of patients often has minimal or no benefits for some, and perhaps many, people who receive it. Consider again the example of intensive cardiac treatment. No one would argue that the growth in intensive cardiac procedures was worthless. But as these procedures have diffused to greater numbers of people, the incremental benefits from further diffusion have declined.

Mark McClellan and colleagues, for example, compared treatment outcomes before and after the beginning of the high-tech revolution in cardiac procedures. They found that the greater likelihood of receiving intensive cardiac care among people living near high-tech hospitals led to only a modest (and possibly no) improvement in health.[16] Along these same lines, the study described in box 2 that found dramatic differences in the use of cardiac procedures across countries found much more modest differences in mortality and morbidity. Put another way, even if the difference in outcomes between a very parsimonious and a moderately generous country (in terms of procedure use) is substantial, the difference between a moderately generous country and a very generous one is not.

The same phenomenon exists for treatment of depression. According to Richard Frank and colleagues, approximately one-quarter of total spending on treatment of depression offers virtually no incremental benefit over nonintervention.[17]

As we elaborate below, the unintended consequences of a handful of public policies are responsible for much of this

relatively wasteful health care spending. The most important flaw in our current policy is the tax preference given
to expenditures financed through insurance. Although there
are a number of exceptions to this rule, the employer-paid
portion of health-insurance costs is generally deductible to
the employer and excludable from the calculation of both
income and payroll taxes by the employee, but out-of-pocket
expenditures must be made from after-tax income.

Economists have long noted two distortionary effects of
this tax preference.[18] First, the exclusion from taxable income
of compensation paid in the form of health insurance makes
buying health care look less expensive to the worker than
its actual cost to society. This observation holds true even
for moderate-income workers with low income-tax rates,
because their employer-provided health insurance is also not
subject to payroll taxes.

Second, the exclusion of compensation paid in the form
of health insurance makes buying health care through insurance instead of out-of-pocket look less expensive to the
worker than it really is. This difference gives people the
incentive to buy their medical care in ways that make them
less conscious of its true cost.

The effect of low-deductible, low-copayment insurance
on use of unproductive health care services has been documented extensively, most notably by the RAND Corporation
in the National Health Insurance Experiment.[19] The RAND
study found that people enrolled in catastrophic health plans
spent only about two-thirds as much on medical care as
those in the full-coverage plan. Equally important, the study
found that health outcomes of those in the catastrophic plans

were, with few exceptions, no different from the outcomes for those in the full-coverage plan.

Various state laws have also contributed to the increasing volume of relatively unproductive expenditures. For example, mandated-benefits laws, which require health plans to cover particular types of persons, services, or providers (such as chiropractic services), increase health-insurance costs by at least 5 percent, and possibly as much as 15 percent.[20] Giving consumers the freedom to choose the benefits package they most prefer would save money and promote more responsible health care spending decisions.

Similarly, "any-willing-provider" laws (which require health plans to accept bills from any doctor, hospital, or pharmacist who is willing to accept the plan's terms and conditions) increase costs by 1–2 percent by weakening the cost-containment effects of managed-care plans.[21] And the most costly states' malpractice systems increase expenditures on "defensive" medicine—treatment based on fear of litigation, which drives up costs but offers minimal health benefits—by approximately 3–7 percent among elderly Medicare beneficiaries with heart disease.[22] While each of these factors increases costs by just a few percentage points, their cumulative effect adds up to billions of dollars each year.

Government health care programs suffer from the same cost problem as the private sector. Since 1970, federal health programs have grown at a 10 percent annual compound rate. Meanwhile, state and local government health care spending has grown at 9 percent per year.[23] The baby boom generation's retirement (the first boomer reaches age 65 next year) will drive government health program costs upward at an even faster rate. Without corrective action, financing public programs will soon require large middle-class tax increases, the issuance of unprecedented amounts of public debt, and large cuts in other programs at all levels of government.

The rapidly rising cost of government health care is, in large part, a consequence of design flaws in public health programs. Medicare was designed as a low-copayment, fee-for-service program to cover a wide range of routine medical services, rather than as a catastrophic health insurance plan. Medicare beneficiaries, with little skin in the game and government picking up the tab, have had little incentive to limit their use of medical services. To control utilization, the government has responded by imposing price controls and other command-and-control regulations on physicians and other health care providers.

The Medicaid program suffers from a similar problem, although its low copayments are understandable given the low incomes of most program beneficiaries. Medicaid has an additional design problem that has contributed to its growth: federal and state governments share the program's costs. Under this shared financing arrangement, each level of government bears only a portion of the cost of any program expansion and receives only a portion of any savings from programmatic reductions. This creates an incentive at the federal level to mandate expansions on all states and for states, in turn, to voluntarily expand benefits which the federal government helps finance. The shared financing also creates disincentives for either level of government to reduce benefits or eligibility. In response to the incentives created by the federal-state matching arrangement, the program continues to grow faster than either level of government would desire if it financed the program solely on its own.

THE UNINSURED POPULATION:
MANY CAUSES, UNCERTAIN CONSEQUENCES

After cost, the number of uninsured is the second-most-frequently expressed concern about health care in the United States. Although the raw number of uninsured—46 million in 2008—is often featured prominently in policy debates, it masks important details that reveal the complexity of the problems of this population.

As box 3 shows, "the uninsured" are composed of three very different groups. The first group, around one-quarter of the uninsured, is already eligible for public insurance, mostly Medicaid, but declines to enroll. For this population, affordability is not the problem: publicly provided insurance is already heavily subsidized. Instead, the problem is likely to involve a broader range of social forces, such as inconvenience, cultural attitudes and stigma, and poor information.[24] Future expansions of public insurance programs like Medicaid are likely to suffer more than past expansions from this "take-up" problem. Take-up was close to complete in the 1980s, before the major Medicaid expansions, but it has fallen considerably over time as more people have become eligible.[25]

The second group, at least another one-quarter, can afford insurance but chooses not to buy it. This group is the fastest-growing of the three. For this relatively affluent group, uninsurance is the inevitable result of rising wasteful spending that does not provide a commensurate increase in value.

Expanding rates of insurance among this population, especially the young and healthy among them, is an important
step in fixing the health care marketplace in America today.
Well-functioning insurance markets require the participation
of large numbers of individuals with widely varying degrees of
health risks. When persons with low risks drop coverage, the
entire insurance market is adversely affected, as their diminished presence in the insurance pool drives up the cost among
those remaining. This outcome can cause the market to break

BOX 3
Who Are the Uninsured?

Estimates of how many Americans are without health insurance
vary widely. Current Population Survey (CPS) data, which measure uninsurance at a point in time during the year, estimate
that approximately 46 million people, or 18 percent of the
nonelderly population, were uninsured in 2008.[26] Many fewer
people were without insurance for an extended period of time.
According to the Survey of Income and Program Participation,
approximately 32 million Americans were uninsured for all
of 2008; according to the Medical Expenditure Panel Survey,
40 million people were uninsured for all of 2008.[27]

"The uninsured" are composed of three distinct groups.
The first group, approximately 12 million people in 2007, are
low-income and eligible for government health-insurance
programs, such as Medicaid and the State Children's Health
Insurance Program (SCHIP), but do not sign up for coverage.[28]
During the 1970s and '80s, the federal and state governments
initiated outreach programs to encourage greater participation. In spite of this, the problem of eligible individuals failing
to enroll continues to plague these programs.

(continued on facing page)

down entirely, as it starts a vicious cycle in which each round of increased costs causes a further exodus of low-risk persons.

For the better-off uninsured, the lack of health insurance is less a failure of private markets that demands government intervention than an example of how public policies have caused the problems we now face. By increasing the cost to workers of employer-provided health insurance, the federal and state tax and regulatory policies previously discussed have had social consequences far beyond their direct finan-

---

(Box 3 *continued*)

The second group, the fastest-growing of the three, is composed of people who can afford health insurance but opt not to buy it. The size of this group depends on what expenditure on insurance is considered "affordable"; according to recent work by Kate Bundorf and Mark Pauly, this group comprises between one-quarter to three-quarters of the uninsured, or 9 to 28 million people.[29] Based on the 2008 Current Population Survey, approximately 10 million uninsured live in households with incomes of $75,000 or more, and 17 million live in households with incomes of $50,000 or more.[30]

The remainder of the uninsured have low or moderate incomes but are not currently eligible for government programs. Some of these individuals, approximately 6 million, are undocumented non-citizens.[31] Others are without insurance for a relatively short period of time. The Congressional Budget Office found that only 18 percent of uninsured individuals with family incomes of less than 200 percent of the poverty line were uninsured for more than two years; 42 percent of uninsured individuals with family incomes of less than 200 percent of the poverty line were uninsured for less than four months.

cial implications. From 2000 to 2010, the average annual cost of an employer-sponsored family insurance policy more than doubled, from $6,438 to $13,770.[32] Just as public policy has the power to generate tremendous benefits when it takes appropriate account of incentives, so does it have the power to generate tremendous costs when it does not.

The number of uninsured is commonly used as an indicator of the problem's severity. Yet, the consequences of being uninsured are not well understood.

Although it may seem surprising, there is little evidence that a lack of health insurance coverage adversely affects a person's health outcomes. Uninsured people obtain significant amounts of medical care—although less than insured people do. According to Jack Hadley and coauthors, medical spending by a full-year uninsured person in 2008 was $1,686, as compared to spending by a full-year privately insured person of $3,915.[33] The effect of this incremental spending—that is, of insurance coverage—on health is at best uncertain. In their comprehensive review of the research on this topic, Helen Levy and David Meltzer conclude that "the central question of how health insurance affects health, for whom it matters, and how much, remains largely unanswered at the level of detail needed to inform policy decision. [M]oreover, for most of the population at risk of being uninsured, we have limited reliable evidence on how health insurance affects health."[34]

Another often-cited consequence of the significant number of uninsured is that insured persons pay higher insurance premiums. According to this reasoning, a significant portion of the costs of treating the uninsured is shifted to the insured through higher premiums. This line of reasoning is often used to argue that tax increases to finance subsidies to cover the uninsured will be recovered through reductions in private insurance premiums.[35]

The empirical basis for this claim is extremely weak. The analyses on this topic that are cited most often, conducted by Families USA and the New America Foundation,[36] have never been subjected to the peer-review process and are seriously flawed. The Families USA analysis is based on statistics that are at odds with other published sources, and the New America Foundation analysis contains numerous conceptual errors.[37] The only recent peer-reviewed study of the cost shift, undertaken by Jack Hadley and coauthors, estimates that the cost shift associated with treating the uninsured raises private health insurance costs by at most 1.7 percent.[38] This magnitude is consistent with work by one of us that finds that cost-shifting in California hospitals raises the cost charged to privately insured patients by 1.4 percent.[39]

The Ugly: Backlash against Markets and the Misguided Policy Response

Over the past twenty years, the dual problems of high costs and uninsurance have given rise to numerous proposals for health reform. Broadly speaking, such proposals have been from two schools of thought. Those from the first school viewed the elimination or reduction of wasteful spending as the primary problem to be addressed. They held that uninsurance—or at least a large part of it—was merely a symptom of the underlying problem of a system of bad incentives. They emphasized market approaches as the solution.

Those from the second school focused on uninsurance. They doubted the usefulness of markets in the context of health care because of imperfect information, individual irrationality, or too little competition. They emphasized the expansion of government as the solution.

THE BACKLASH AGAINST MARKETS

Ironically, the nation's experience with managed care in the 1990s galvanized support for this perspective. Managed care was, at least in part, the solution markets offered to the problem of relatively unproductive health care expenditures induced by policy. Health care experts widely agree that managed care played a central role in slowing medical expenditure growth during the 1990s. In response to the incentives provided by managed care, providers curtailed the growth in spending on enrollees. In addition, competition from managed-care plans forced conventional private insurers and public insurance programs to reduce the growth in spending.[40]

But managed care failed to change the incentives that underlay individual patients' demands for health care services and, as a result, enrollees continued to demand high levels of service. When high demand met curtailed supply, a backlash against markets was the result. In 2003, Americans rated managed-care and health-insurance companies more unfavorably than every other industry (see figure 2).[41] Fully 52 percent of people polled said that the government needed

FIGURE 2

Health Care Is the Most Negatively Perceived Sector

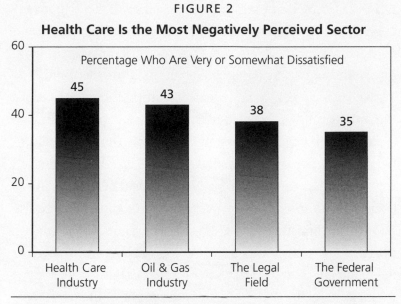

Source: "Survey Results on Cost of Health Care and Health Insurance," Market Strategies Inc.

to protect consumers from being treated unfairly and not getting the care they should from managed-care plans.[42]

THE MISGUIDED POLICY RESPONSE

Proposals from the second school culminated in the Patient Protection and Affordable Care Act—the most significant health reform since Medicare—signed into law by President Obama on March 23, 2010. The law's primary focus is to increase insurance coverage. According to the Congressional Budget Office, it will cut the percentage of uninsured from 18 percent today to 8 percent in 2016.[43]

It seeks to accomplish this goal in three ways. It mandates that citizens and legal residents buy, and that employers offer, health insurance or pay tax penalties; it creates a major new entitlement to subsidize the purchase of the newly mandated private insurance; it creates another entitlement for long-term care; and it vastly expands eligibility for Medicaid.

The law also expands federal insurance regulation. In the individual and small-group markets, it will require insurance companies to cover all persons who apply (termed "guaranteed issue"), charge all persons in the same age-gender group the same premiums regardless of their health status (termed community rating), and prevent or inhibit insurance companies from raising copayments. It will require that health plans cover "essential health benefits" (to be defined by the Secretary of Health and Human Services) and standardize their offerings into at most four types of plans that must meet minimum actuarial value standards. The law also imposes numerous new regulations on other employer-sponsored health plans; we discuss the consequences of these regulations, and suggest potential reforms to them, in chapter 2.

Without question, the law will increase the nation's spending on health care. As the research by Jack Hadley and coauthors discussed above shows, the typical insured person spends more than twice as much on health care as the typical uninsured person. The increase in the number of persons covered by health insurance, estimated by CBO to be near 30 million, will add significantly to aggregate health care spending. Second, because the supply of physicians and other inputs to the production of health services are fixed in the short to medium run, this expansion of demand will increase costs for the existing privately insured population. We calculate that health insurance premiums for the typical family plan will rise by about 10 percent as a result of the coverage expansion.[44] Because an employer-sponsored family insurance plan cost $13,770 in 2010, this translates into an increase of approximately $1,400 in the typical annual premium. In addition, as we show in greater detail in chapter 2, the expansion of insurance regulation will further increase insurance costs for both the newly insured and the already insured.

There is no provision in the law of corresponding importance that seeks to control costs. The most promising provision is the law's limit on the current open-ended tax exclusion for employer-sponsored insurance. Starting in 2018, the new law proposes to establish an excise tax of 40 percent on high-cost health plans. In an ideal world, such a tax would effectively repeal the exclusion for spending on health insurance above a certain amount. However, as we discuss in greater detail in chapter 2, there are several reasons to doubt the effectiveness of the tax change.

The negative effects of the law, however, reach beyond its failure to deal with the cost problem. Because the law must specify the parameters of the insurance policies that can be bought with its new subsidies, it shifts control of coverage decisions from markets to government—and so drives a new wedge between individuals' health care arrangements and their preferences.

As the new health care law drives health insurance premiums upward, there will undoubtedly be renewed calls for a "public option." As its name implies, the public option would create a government-owned and controlled health plan that would operate in the same market as private insurance plans. Such a plan would offer persons seeking insurance an alternative to existing private plans.

The public option would fail to solve any of the significant problems created by the recently enacted health care law, and it would exacerbate many others. The government plan would contain low copayments and broad coverage similar to the mandated health plans under the new law. In addition, the political control inherent in a public plan will result in reimbursement rates that reflect, at least in part, the relative political power of different constituencies.[45] Such a government-administered pricing scheme will have important consequences for consumers. Services that are underpriced will become scarce, and patients will experience longer waiting times to receive treatment. Services that are overpriced will become abundant as providers are induced to supply more than is medically necessary. Finally, the government plan would receive generous taxpayer-financed subsidies that would allow it to undercut its private competitors and expand, even if it offered no advantages to consumers. As unsubsidized private health plans exit the market, health insurance choices available to consumers would decline. In the worst case, only the government plan would remain, and the U.S. health care market would have evolved into a government-run single-payer system.[46]

The law also promises to have negative effects on the broader U.S. economy. First, despite claims to the contrary, the law will lead to some combination of greater deficits and higher taxes. According to the Congressional Budget Office, the new health care entitlements will raise federal health care spending by nearly $1 trillion during the next ten years.[47] The funds to pay for it come largely from two sources: cuts to Medicare reimbursement and new taxes.[48]

The reductions in Medicare reimbursement rates are unlikely to be sustained. For the past twenty-five years, Congress has repeatedly promised to "cut" Medicare reimbursement rates, with limited (if any) success. The problem is that long-term reimbursement rate cuts rarely deliver the savings that they promise because of the ability of providers and future Congresses to undo them. Indeed, at the same time Congress was claiming Medicare savings to finance the new law, it was undoing Medicare savings that were achieved by another law: on April 15, 2010, less than a month after the new law was passed, President Obama signed a bill that prevented a scheduled cut in physician reimbursements. The budget impact from this action had no effect on the CBO's scoring of the health plan because it was written into another law.

Second, the new law will have far-reaching negative effects on rewards to work. The law's generous private insurance subsidies phase out as income rises. This phase-out rate can run as high as 50 percent; that is, for each dollar of additional earnings, the amount of the federal subsidy can decline by as much as 50 cents.[49] This implicit tax comes on top of existing income and payroll taxes. For many middle-income families, the combined impact of the phase-out and existing state and federal taxes raises the effective marginal tax rates on earnings to around 80–100 percent.[50] Tax rates this high will destroy most of the income gains from additional work, skill development, or job promotion for a broad cross-section of middle-income workers, which will inevitably have a significant labor market impact.

Third, the law's mandate that some employers must provide health insurance or pay a penalty will create other distortions. Because the law exempts from the mandate firms with employment levels below a certain threshold, it creates an incentive for employers to reduce their workforces.[51] For firms with employment levels above the threshold, the mandate raises the cost of full-time labor.[52] This higher cost cannot be offset by lowering wages paid to workers at or just above the minimum wage. As empirical research on the effect of a health insurance mandate has shown, the consequences of an effective increase in the minimum wage of this magnitude will be increased unemployment.[53]

CHAPTER 2

Five Policy Reforms
to Make Markets Work

Although America's health care system is strong in many respects, poorly designed public policies have created significant problems as well—relatively unproductive care; a growing number of people without health insurance; an increase in bureaucratic controls with a corresponding loss of personal and medical authority; and an excessive number of medical errors. Many interpret these problems as evidence that individual choice and markets are the wrong way to deliver health care. The problem, though, is not that market forces cannot work in health care. Rather, public policies have prevented health care markets from functioning properly.

The tax preference for employer health insurance has created a health care system in which doctors and patients bear few of the resource costs of their decisions. This system was grafted onto government health care programs. In this perverse world, true insurance, in the form of coverage for catastrophic health events, is the exception; prepaid health care, in the form of coverage with low deductibles and copayments, is the rule.

The pervasiveness of prepaid health care instead of true insurance, in turn, encourages the consumption of relatively unproductive care. Inefficient regulation and one-size-fits-all government health care programs prevent people from purchasing the type of insurance that they want. In addition, the malpractice system has both encouraged wasteful expenditures and discouraged investment in addressing the problem of medical errors.

When combined with technological improvements, these policies inevitably lead to rising costs. In response, the system has sought to limit cost growth through the use of administrative controls such as gatekeepers, rather than cost-conscious consumers. The overuse of gatekeepers has had numerous and potentially profound adverse effects— the direct cost of the extra gatekeepers; the loss of consumer decision-making authority; and the damage to the prospects of developing effective public policies caused by the public perception that markets do not work in health care.

Despite the shortcomings of current policy, the infrastructure for improving the functioning of markets is nonetheless in place. Flexible spending accounts and health savings accounts allow consumers to incorporate more of the true treatment costs in their decisions.

Five policy changes would further promote more efficient purchasing of medical care, stimulate a vigorous, competitive market for insurance, expand coverage of the currently uninsured, and reduce medical errors:

1. Encourage greater individual involvement in health care decisions by changing the tax law to reduce the preference for medical-care purchases through employer-sponsored health insurance and by increasing cost-sharing in government programs.

2. Deregulate insurance markets and redesign government programs.

3. Expand provision of health information.

4. Control anticompetitive behavior by providers and insurers.

5. Reform the malpractice system.

Finally, we propose that a sixth potential reform be studied further: revocation or limitation of the current tax preference for nonprofits.

Increase Individual Involvement in Health Care Decisions

The fundamental cause of the high cost of health care in the United States is that individuals and providers lack incentives to limit the use of medical services. Because most health care is paid for through low-deductible, low-coinsurance health plans, individuals pay only a small fraction of the costs of the care they receive and have too little skin in the game. The lack of incentives is also pervasive in government programs. The paths by which private plans and government programs have created this fundamental problem, though different, can be traced back to a handful of misguided public policies. Modifying these policies will go a long way toward reducing health care costs without impairing innovation and the quality of medical care.

IN PRIVATE MARKETS, REFORM TAXATION OF HEALTH SPENDING

Preferential treatment of employer-paid health insurance costs by public policy began with a seemingly innocuous provision of the Stabilization Act of 1942, which limited the wage increases that employers could grant but permitted employer-paid health insurance to be provided as a fringe benefit exempt from wage controls. The preference was extended to the tax code shortly thereafter. Under a 1943 administrative tax-court ruling and 1954 changes to the Internal Revenue Code, employer contributions to employee health-insurance costs became deductible to the employer and nontaxable to the employee.[1]

This tax preference has never been absolute, however. Extraordinary medical expenses paid out-of-pocket have long been deductible to varying degrees. Under the Revenue Act of 1942, medical expenses in excess of 5 percent of a taxpayer's adjusted gross income, up to $2,500, qualified as an itemized deduction.[2] The floor for the medical-expense deduction was lowered to 3 percent (and the ceiling was raised) in 1954; the floor was raised back to 5 percent in

1982, raised again to 7.5 percent 1986, and raised to 10 percent by the PPACA.[3]

The tax preference has created a strong financial incentive for individuals to purchase medical care through employer-provided insurance. Neither employer nor employee pays income or payroll taxes on the employer's contribution to an employee's insurance plan. By contrast, a worker who purchases health insurance on his own must finance the purchase with after-tax income—that is, income that remains after income and payroll taxes have been deducted. A typical middle-income worker faces a marginal federal income tax rate of 15 percent and a payroll tax rate on wages of 7.65 percent. An employer must also pay a payroll tax of 7.65 percent on wages, raising the total marginal tax rate on wage income to approximately 30 percent.

By purchasing health insurance through the employer, these taxes are avoided; together, the employer and employee save almost one-third of the cost of a health care plan compared to having the employee purchase medical care or health insurance on his own. At least in part due to the tax preference, 176 million out of 201 million persons who are covered by private health insurance are enrolled in employer-sponsored plans.[4]

Similarly, the tax preference has also created large incentives to purchase employer-provided insurance with low deductibles and copayment rates, even though such plans cost considerably more than catastrophic health insurance. Several studies conclude that revoking the tax preference for employer-provided insurance would lead the effective coinsurance rate to double.[5] For employers, this change would translate into average premiums for group health insurance that were 45 percent lower.[6]

These estimates are consistent with other evidence. According to unpublished data for 2003 from Anthem, a large health insurer now part of WellPoint, the average annual deductible among plans purchased through large firms (500 or more employees), and hence excluded from taxation, was $250; the average deductible among plans purchased directly by individuals, most of which were purchased with after-tax income, was $1,250, or five times greater.[7]

Health plans with low deductibles and coinsurance rates create a "moral hazard" that leads patients and their physicians to use too many services that do little to improve measurable health outcomes. According to the RAND Corporation's National Health Insurance Experiment, an increase in a health plan's annual deductible from $200 to $500 reduces the total amount an individual spends on health care through both insurance and out-of-pocket payments by nearly 5 percent.[8]

Similarly, an increase in a plan's coinsurance rate from 25 to 35 percent reduces the total amount an individual spends on health care services by approximately 8 percent.[9] Although these percentages might seem small, when aggregated over the entire population with private health insurance, the impact is large. Each percentage-point increase in health care spending among this group equals $7 billion a year. And, these changes occur without any appreciable impact on most individuals' measurable health outcomes.[10]

In a recent paper, we estimate the effect of the tax preference for insurance on health spending based on the Medical

Expenditure Panel Surveys (MEPS) from 1996–2005.[11] We use the fact that Social Security taxes are only levied on earnings below a statutory threshold to identify the tax preference's impact. Because employer-sponsored health insurance premiums are excluded from Social Security payroll taxes, workers who earn just below the Social Security tax threshold receive a larger tax preference for health insurance than workers who earn just above it.

We find a significant effect of the tax preference. Depending on the specification of our model, we estimate that repealing the tax preference would reduce health spending by people with employer-sponsored insurance by between 26 and 33 percent. These estimates, while quite large, are consistent with previous research. Using a proprietary simulation model, for example, Jonathan Gruber calculates that repealing all tax subsidies for health insurance would result in a 43 percent decline in health spending.[12]

Thus, the tax preference for buying medical care through employer-sponsored insurance is largely responsible for creating today's health-insurance market, in which third parties pay five out of every six dollars spent on medical-care services, and individual consumers and health care providers exhibit little cost consciousness. Elected officials, however, have been unwilling to eliminate the tax exclusion for employer-provided insurance, presumably because it would significantly raise taxes on a broad class of taxpayers.

To make this point clear, consider a household facing a combined marginal income-tax and payroll-tax rate of 30 percent. Suppose that the household's employer makes a $6,600 annual contribution to the household's health-insurance plan.[13] Repealing the tax exclusion would increase this household's taxes by approximately $2,000. Higher-income households with employer-sponsored insurance would have their taxes raised by more, and lower-income households would have their taxes raised by less. But all 175 million persons who are covered by employer-sponsored insurance would have taxes on their wage compensation increased.

There have been numerous attempts to limit the health-insurance tax exclusion in the past thirty years. President Reagan expressed a willingness to consider it in 1983. That year he proposed to cap the amount of employer-provided insurance that could be excluded from taxation. His proposal was soundly rejected in Congress. A similar proposal was considered and rejected during the 1985 tax-reform debate. In 2005, President George W. Bush proposed to replace the insurance tax exclusion with a $15,000 tax deduction, effectively capping the exclusion at $15,000. His proposal failed to attract any serious attention in Congress. More recently, 2008 presidential candidate John McCain proposed eliminating the exclusion and replacing it with a tax credit.

As we noted in chapter 1, despite intense opposition, the Patient Protection and Affordable Care Act put an end to the unlimited tax exclusion. Starting in 2018, the new law proposes to establish an excise tax of 40 percent on high cost health plans. Whether this tax will ultimately be allowed to take effect is highly uncertain. Even if the tax becomes effective, its numerous loopholes lead us to question just how effective it will be in eliminating the tax bias that favors health insurance over out-of-pocket payments.

An alternative approach to removing the tax bias that favors health insurance over out-of-pocket payments is to exclude from taxation out-of-pocket payments. In contrast to the extension of taxation to employer-sponsored insurance, this policy takes the approach that Congress has used successfully since the late 1970s.

First, changes in 1978 to Section 125 of the Internal Revenue Code allowed expenditures made through an employer's "cafeteria" plan to be deductible to the employer but nontaxable to the employee. Such "flexible spending accounts" allow employees to allocate a portion of their compensation to nontaxable fringe benefits instead of taxable wages. Currently, once the amount of the contribution has been designated, the employee is not allowed to change it or drop the plan during the year unless he or she experiences a change of family status. By law, the employee forfeits any unspent funds in the account at the end of the year.[14]

This result has the unfortunate effect of creating incentives for individuals who have unspent funds near year's end to consume more health care services simply to avoid forfeiting the funds. Prior to Treasury Department regulations issued in 1984, there was no such "use-it-or-lose-it" provision implied by Section 125, making the cafeteria-plan exception even more generous to employees.[15]

Second, under Treasury regulations issued in 2002, sections 105 and 106 of the Internal Revenue Code allow "health-reimbursement arrangements," also known as "health-reimbursement accounts" or "personal-care accounts," to reimburse employees for medical expenses with before-tax dollars, without the use-it-or-lose-it provision of Section 125 cafeteria plans.[16]

Third, under the Medicare Prescription Drug, Improvement, and Modernization Act of 2003, employers and individuals with qualifying health insurance plans can make tax-free contributions to health savings accounts. Funds from these accounts can be used to pay for medical expenses in the present or the future. However, the fact that qualifying plans must have very high deductibles has limited the take-up of these accounts.

We propose to build on this approach by making three simple changes in tax policy to promote more efficient insurance policy design, to offer incentives for consumers to be better shoppers, and to enhance tax fairness. These changes are the allowance of full deductibility of health care expenses, modified health savings accounts, and tax credits for low-income households.

Full Deductibility of Health Expenses. All Americans should be entitled to deduct expenditures on health insurance and out-of-pocket health care expenses as long as they purchase insurance that covers at least catastrophic expenditures. That is, individuals already covered by employer-sponsored insurance may deduct out-of-pocket expenses and their employee contributions. Self-employed individuals with insurance may deduct out-of-pocket expenses. Individuals currently without coverage may deduct insurance premiums and out-of-pocket expenses if they choose to purchase an insurance plan. (In all cases, the deduction is "above the line"—available even to taxpayers not itemizing income-tax deductions.)[17]

Allowing direct individual payments for health care to be tax-deductible promotes insurance that provides financial protection from catastrophic illness or injury, and yet creates significant incentives for individuals to be cost-conscious in their decisions about health care. We call such insurance "true" insurance. The policy does so by reducing the tax bias against out-of-pocket health expenditures.

Under the current tax treatment, any medical care purchased through employer-sponsored insurance is paid for with pretax dollars, while care purchased out of pocket is paid for with after-tax dollars. Recall from our previous example that, even for a middle-income family, the differential is substantial, amounting to approximately 30 percent when both federal income and payroll taxes are considered. Once the tax bias is reduced, individuals will find it in their financial interest to purchase health plans with lower premiums and higher copayments (see box 4), a shift that will give them incentives to make careful choices about their health care spending, as well as the opportunity to save money.

In addition, allowing direct health care expenses to be tax-deductible will significantly reduce the growth in health costs, as greater cost consciousness leads to less spending. Below, we show that for any plausible set of parameter values, this curtailment of spending will more than offset any increase in out-of-pocket spending that occurs because tax-deductibility lowers the cost of health care spending compared to other goods.

BOX 4
How Full Deductibility Promotes Cost-Conscious Insurance

Consider a family that expects to spend $3,600 on health care in the coming year and is concerned that it could end up spending a lot more. Suppose the family's employer offers a choice between a health plan with a high annual premium ($5,400) that requires no deductible and a plan with a lower annual premium ($3,000) that has a deductible of $1,800. For simplicity, assume that the coinsurance rate for expenses above the deductible is zero. If the family chooses the latter plan, the employer will increase the family's salary income by the amount of the premium savings, less the additional payroll taxes the employer is required to withhold (7.65 percent).

Under current tax law, the family will choose the zero-deductible plan. If the family chooses the $1,800-deductible plan, it will receive $2,216 from the employer (the premium

(continued on facing page)

Our proposal for full deductibility has several other beneficial effects. Deductibility mitigates the bias against individual insurance because both employer-sponsored and individual insurance can be acquired with pre–income tax dollars. However, because the tax change allows the deduction of the cost of individual insurance from the income-tax base but not from the payroll-tax base, the proposed policy retains a significant tax incentive for the purchase of employer-sponsored insurance. Expenditures on insurance purchased through an employer would, as under current law, still be excludable from both the income-tax and payroll-tax bases.

(Box 4 *continued*)

savings of $2,400, less the employer's share of payroll taxes of $184). But because the family is required to pay an additional $502 in income and payroll taxes (= $2,216 × 15 percent federal income tax plus 7.65 percent payroll tax), it receives only $1,714. This total is $86 less than the expected increase in the family's out-of-pocket expenditures under the $1,800-deductible plan.

If out-of-pocket expenses were tax-deductible, however, the family would choose the $1,800-deductible plan. The family would realize a tax savings of $270 (= $1,800 × 15 percent federal income tax) from its higher out-of-pocket health care spending under the $1,800-deductible plan. Thus, its net tax burden would rise by only $232 (= $502 − $270) instead of $502.

The family's after-tax income would, therefore, rise by $1,984 ($2,216 − $232). This increase is $184 more than the expected increase in the family's out-of-pocket expenditures under the $1,800-deductible plan.

Because the tax change allows the deductibility of out-of-pocket health care expenses only with the purchase of insurance, the proposed policy also creates a significant tax incentive for the currently uninsured to purchase insurance. Under current law, a typical uninsured person receives no tax benefit from purchasing coverage. Under our proposal, an individual who purchased a $2,000 health plan and also paid $1,000 in out-of-pocket expenses would not only be able to deduct the cost of out-of-pocket expenses, but also his health-insurance premiums. Indeed, for a person in the 15 percent tax bracket, the tax deduction is worth $450—23 percent of the cost of insurance.

The tax change also enhances the fairness of the federal income-tax system. Under current law, individuals whose employers decline to offer them insurance are penalized because they must purchase it with after-tax income. Tax deductibility would promote simplicity by replacing the myriad of currently available special health care deductions previously discussed with a single deduction equally applicable to all individuals. Finally, as we show below, deductibility would also increase the progressivity of the tax system. Although marginal tax rates are higher for higher-income people, the fact that lower-income people have higher (currently taxable) out-of-pocket spending more than compensates for this effect.

On this dimension, the Patient Protection and Affordable Care Act unfortunately moves tax policy in the opposite direction. First, effective in 2013, it caps contributions to Section 125 flexible spending accounts at $2,500 per year. Second, it proposes to count contributions to flexible spending accounts toward the spending cap on which the 40 percent excise tax is based. Third, it increases the threshold for the itemized deduction for unreimbursed medical expenses, from 7.5 percent to 10 percent of adjusted gross income.

Finally, it provides means-tested subsidies not only for premiums but also for copayments. This change has the perverse effect of purposefully dampening individuals' incentives to consider the true cost of health care. For any given level of subsidy, beneficiaries could be made better off by giving them the entire subsidy in the form of a credit against premiums, and letting them decide which copayment structure would best suit their needs.

Modified Health Savings Accounts. The tax code can also be changed to make it easier for individuals and families to save for expenses not covered by higher-deductible insurance. Medical savings accounts (MSAs) and health savings accounts (HSAs) currently permit tax-free contributions for individuals purchasing high-deductible health-insurance plans. We propose making all individuals eligible for health savings accounts, conditional on the purchase of insurance that covers at least catastrophic expenditures. As with current HSAs, balances may be spent on the health care of a relative, and balances not spent on health care could be carried forward tax-free. Funds withdrawn for purposes other than health care would be subject to income tax. Recipients of health care tax credits (described below) could deposit funds in a health savings account, if they wished.

We propose three significant changes to HSAs. First, under current law, an employer-sponsored family health-insurance plan must have a deductible of at least $1,200 to qualify its purchaser for the HSA ($2,400 for a family). We would eliminate the minimum deductible requirement. Second, for persons under age fifty-five, the annual amount a person can deposit in an HSA is currently limited to a maximum of $3,050 ($6,150 for a family). Since our plan will make all current health care expenses tax deductible, the role of HSAs will be to enable tax-free saving for future health care needs. To maintain parity with current law, we would allow individuals to save tax-free the difference between the current HSA maximum deposit and the current minimum required deductible, which is about $1,800 for an individual and $3,700 for a family. Third, under current law, funds from an HSA cannot be used to purchase insurance. Under our proposal, funds from an HSA can be used for any qualified health care expense.

The purpose of these proposed changes is to make the HSA law less prescriptive and, thereby, to encourage greater use of HSAs. We are concerned that the high-deductible requirement under current law may serve as an important barrier to widespread use of HSAs. Under our proposal, individuals would be free to choose the deductible level, make tradeoffs between the deductible and coinsurance amounts, and purchase insurance on their own rather than through an employer, all without tax penalty. Consistent with our policy of full deductibility, we believe that public policy should, whenever possible, allow individual preferences rather than government mandates to determine people's health-insurance arrangements.

Tax Credits for Low-Income Households. A third policy we support is designed to improve the health care "safety net" for low-income households. While our proposal to make out-of-pocket medical expenses tax-deductible offers important benefits for many low- and middle-income working families, it does not help families that pay little or no income tax.

To offer low-income households financial assistance to purchase health care, we propose a tax credit, applicable against income or payroll taxes, that would subsidize 25 percent of health expenses up to a maximum of $1,000 for an individual ($2,000 for a family). Health care expenses would include both payments for insurance and out-of-pocket expenses. Thus, the credit would be available to buy insurance through an employer, on one's own, or to pay for out-of-pocket expenses (conditional on having insurance).

The full subsidy should be available to households with income below the poverty level. The subsidy would be gradually phased out for households with incomes between 100 and 300 percent of the poverty level. Households could not claim both the tax deduction for direct medical expenses and the tax credit, but instead would be required to choose between the two.

This credit structure has two desirable features. First, it can be applied toward any health expense—insured or out-of-pocket—and so does not create a tax preference for insurance. Second, the amount of the tax credit is limited to the household's tax liability, and so the policy avoids creating a new, open-ended entitlement.

Our tax-reform policies will encourage people to substitute true insurance for their current prepaid health care arrangements. These policies enhance the incentives for people to use their own out-of-pocket payments or savings rather than third parties to finance ordinary health expenses. This substitution will lead health costs and, in turn, rates of uninsurance to decline. At the same time, these policies enhance the incentives for uninsured people to purchase insurance, make the tax system fairer, and offer a direct benefit to low- and middle-income people to help them meet rising health costs. Collectively, by reducing the current tax bias against low-cost catastrophic insurance, these policies will help develop a more robust market for such insurance. Box 5 summarizes the tax benefits for the purchase of health insurance in our proposals.

BOX 5
Tax Benefits for the Purchase of Health Insurance, Current and Proposed Law

	Current Law	Proposed Law
Individuals with Employer-Sponsored Insurance	Employer-paid premiums excluded from income and payroll taxes; out-of-pocket expenses and employee premium payments not deductible unless employer has a Section 125 plan. Individuals with high-deductible insurance plans can make limited tax-free contributions to health savings accounts. Individuals working for employers with a Section 125 plan can make "use-it-or-lose-it" contributions, capped at $2,500 starting in 2013.	Employer-paid premiums continue to be excluded from both income and payroll taxation; out-of-pocket expenses and employee premium payments would be deductible from income taxes, but not payroll taxes. Premiums continue to be deductible from income but not payroll taxes; out-of-pocket expenses deductible if person is covered by insurance. Tax-free contributions to health savings accounts of $1,800 ($3,700 for families) could be made regardless of the health plan's deductible level. Health care tax credit covering 25 percent of health care insurance and out-of-pocket expenses up to $1,000 ($2,000 for families).
Self-Employed	Premiums deductible for purposes of income but not payroll taxes; out-of-pocket expenses generally not deductible. Deductibility of health savings accounts as above.	Premiums continue to be deductible from income but not payroll taxes; out-of-pocket expenses deductible if person is covered by insurance. Tax-free contributions to health savings accounts of $1,800 ($3,700 for families) could be made regardless of the health plan's deductible level. Health care tax credit covering 25 percent of health care insurance and out-of-pocket expenses up to $1,000 ($2,000 for families).
All Others	Neither premiums nor out-of-pocket expenses are generally deductible.	

INCREASE COST SHARING IN GOVERNMENT PROGRAMS

Medicare. The Medicare program's design was based on the structure of private sector health plans in existence at the time of the program's creation in 1965. By this time, the health insurance tax exclusion had been in operation for two decades and its impact was reflected in the high prevalence of low-deductible, low-coinsurance health plans in the private sector. Thus, Medicare, instead of being based on true insurance principles and protecting against the risk of catastrophic loss, was originally designed as a program with low copayments and low coinsurance. In effect, by using existing private sector plans as its model, Medicare's original design incorporated the same fundamental flaws that the tax code had created for private sector plans.

Subsequent legislative changes over the past forty-five years have reduced copayments from these initially low levels. For example, in the late 1980s the federal government limited the freedom of physicians to charge patients for Medicare services and eliminated balance billing almost entirely in the early 1990s. Today, Medicare limits copayments to zero for laboratory tests and home health services, and only 20 percent for physician services and medical equipment. Similarly, for decades, the federal government failed to allow the deductible charged for Medicare Part B (outpatient) services to rise with health care costs. As a result, since 1965, although medical care costs have risen to fourteen times their original level, the Medicare Part B deductible has only risen from $50 to $162, an approximately three-fold increase.

The combined impact of these actions on Medicare Part B cost sharing has been significant. In 1977, Medicare

Part B copayments in the form of payments to meet the plan's deductible, coinsurance, and payments to physicians under balance-billing arrangements accounted for 37 percent of total Part B payments.[18] In 2008, these payments accounted for 21 percent, just over half of their 1977 level.[19]

Unfortunately, physician and other outpatient services are precisely those for which utilization is most responsive to copayments.[20] At least in part as a result of these low copayments, increasing utilization of medical services per recipient, rather than the rising number of Medicare beneficiaries or medical care inflation, has been the driving force behind Medicare's expenditure growth.[21]

The Medicare program, like private sector health insurance, needs to be restructured to encourage individuals to use their own out-of-pocket payments or savings to finance their routine health care expenses. Medicare recipients, like their younger counterparts who have private health insurance, need to have more skin in the game. In return, Medicare should be expanded to offer individuals greater protection against the high costs of catastrophic illness. Currently, Medicare has no limit to the amount individuals pay out-of-pocket for hospital and physician care.

The magnitude of savings in health care costs from higher copayments ultimately depends on the responsiveness of senior citizens' health care consumption to higher copayments. Although no precise estimates of their responses exist, there are good reasons to believe that the savings may be substantial. To illustrate, suppose copayments for Medicare Part B were raised from their current level (approximately 20 percent) to the level that prevailed in the mid-1970s (approximately 40 percent). If Medicare beneficiaries' response to copayments were the same as the privately insured non-elderly, then taxpayer-financed Medicare Part B expenditures would decline by 38 percent.[22] Even if the beneficiaries' response were *only half* that of persons under age 65, taxpayer-financed expenditures would decline by 29 percent.[23]

One way that has been proposed to achieve this outcome is to give Medicare beneficiaries a risk-adjusted payment (for example, an amount that varies with the individual's health status) with which to purchase a health plan, choosing from a menu that includes a plan with significantly more cost sharing.[24] As we discuss below, we support this approach, but because political barriers make its adoption in the near-term unlikely, we also offer a short-term solution: expand traditional Medicare to include a plan with greater cost-sharing. Such a change could build on the new Medicare Medical Savings Account (MSA) Plans that were first offered to beneficiaries in 2007.

To encourage beneficiaries to choose such a plan, we propose sharing the gains from it with them in three ways. First, the plan could include catastrophic protection in the form of maximum limits on total out-of-pocket expenses for covered services or greater nursing home coverage as Medicare MSA plans do. Second, the premiums for the plan could be set below those charged for the current Medicare Part B program. Third, beneficiaries who opt for the plan could be allowed to contribute to health savings accounts, which under current law they are precluded from doing.

Medicaid. The objective of raising copayments should also be applied to the Medicaid program. The low incomes of Medicaid beneficiaries, of course, limit the extent to which this can be done. However, this constraint can be addressed by providing beneficiaries with additional cash assistance to offset the financial impact of higher copayments. The cash assistance would be a fixed amount that would be allowed to vary depending on the person's health status. Since most Medicaid recipients also simultaneously receive some regular cash assistance from government welfare programs, the supplemental monthly payments can be made with little or no added administrative burden.[25]

Deregulate Insurance Markets and Redesign Medicare and Medicaid

Getting individuals more involved in their health care decisions is necessary, but not sufficient, to obtain better value for the country's health care dollar. Changes to the supply side of the market must also occur to enable the demand-side reforms previously detailed to work. In private markets, we need to remove benefits mandates and other regulations that discourage or prevent private markets from offering cost-conscious options. We also need to change the fundamental structure of public programs to increase the extent to which they adapt to participants' preferences while evolving in a fiscally sustainable way.

DEREGULATE INSURANCE MARKETS

Under the McCarran-Ferguson Act, state governments had primary responsibility for regulating health-insurance markets. Each state specified the rules by which its insurance market operated, including the financial requirements insurers must meet in order to sell policies in the state, the particular services that a health-insurance plan must cover, the prices insurers can charge, the individuals or groups that must be offered coverage, and the method by which insurance companies must conduct their business operations. Until the enactment of the PPACA, the federal government played only a limited role. The main law, the Employee Retirement and Income Security Act (ERISA) of 1974, exempted self-insured employer-sponsored health care plans from many of these costly state regulations.[26]

Unfortunately, states have used their authority in ways that have been harmful to well-functioning markets. For example, New York requires insurance companies to offer coverage at the same price to all persons in a given age and gender group regardless of health status. Such community-rating rules increase premiums and reduce insurance coverage. Previous empirical research has found that the large, implicit transfer that community rating creates causes relatively healthy people to drop out of the market, leading premiums to rise for those who remain.[27]

Many states also require that specific benefits and providers be covered by all health-insurance plans. In 1965, there were less than a dozen such mandates in laws throughout the fifty states and the District of Columbia; by 2009, the number had risen to over 2,100.[28] For example, California requires insurance plans to cover both contraceptives and in-vitro fertilization; Virginia requires coverage of contraceptives but not in-vitro fertilization; and Florida, Indiana, and Pennsylvania require coverage of neither service.[29]

Some states also adopted laws, termed "any-willing-provider" laws, that require health plans to reimburse expenses for care provided by any doctor, hospital, or pharmacist who is willing to accept the plans' terms and conditions. Such laws stifle health plans' ability to require providers to compete with one another to improve quality and contain costs.

States' mandated benefits and rate regulations have driven up the cost of insurance significantly. Mandates have raised the cost of a typical insurance plan by at least 5 percent and possibly as much as 15 percent.[30] Any-willing-provider laws drive up health care costs by as much as 1.8 percent.[31] In turn, the rising costs imposed by benefits mandates and regulation have reduced the number of persons with health insurance. Although there is considerable uncertainty about the precise magnitude of the reduction, one study estimates about 25 percent of the people who are without health insurance are uninsured because of the cost of state mandates alone.[32]

In contrast to the states, the federal government imposed only minimal regulations on private insurance prior to the enactment of the Patient Protection and Affordable Care Act. Self-insured health plans governed by ERISA, for example, have been free to offer a health benefit plan largely of their choosing.[33] The freedom from heavy state regulation is one reason why more than half of all employees in employer-sponsored plans in 2008 were enrolled in ERISA plans subject to federal, as opposed to state, regulation.[34]

The passage of the PPACA alters this landscape by significantly expanding the federal regulation of health insurance markets.[35] Key regulations that apply to all health plans, whether they are self-insured or fully insured, include bans on the exclusion of pre-existing conditions from coverage; bans on annual and lifetime limits on "essential" health benefits; and mandates that family insurance plans offer coverage to adult children under 26 years of age. Key regulations that apply to insured plans only include the requirement that insurers community-rate their premiums and sell to all persons who request coverage;[36] limits on the cost-sharing that plans can offer;[37] and restrictions on medical loss ratios.[38] In addition, the new law requires insurers to participate in risk-adjustment programs that each state must establish (in which plans with relatively healthier enrollees make payments to plans with relatively sicker enrollees) and establishes a temporary "reinsurance" fund to subsidize insurers with sicker-than-expected enrollees, financed with a tax on all health insurance and employer-sponsored health insured plans.

On the whole, the new law moves insurance regulation in the wrong direction. Most important, its community-rating provisions, as we previously noted, will raise insurance premiums and reduce insurance coverage. Its limits on cost-sharing and medical loss ratios have the effect of enshrining into law the very features of health insurance at the root of the market's fundamental problem: incentives for generous coverage without regard to the moral hazard it creates.[39]

Our research on the effects of health reform in Massachusetts suggests that the overall impact of the law will be to raise private insurance premiums. Because the Massachusetts reform's main components are similar to those of the new federal law, the consequences of the

Massachusetts reform offer a window onto potential national impact. Although this research does not disentangle the effect of the regulatory aspects of the Massachusetts reform from other potential effects, we find that the Massachusetts reform increased employer-sponsored insurance premiums there by approximately 6 percent.[40]

Our proposed policy consists of two reforms to regulation of insurance markets: allow insurers to offer plans on a nationwide basis, free from costly state benefit mandates and regulation; and subsidize the costs of caring for persistently high-cost, chronically ill patients.

Foster Nationwide, Portable Health Insurance. The key objective of insurance reform is to improve the availability and portability of low-cost health insurance. This can be best accomplished by creating a nationwide insurance market. Such a market should allow individuals to buy insurance plans that are free of provider and benefit mandates and to retain their plans when they move from state to state.

This approach would make insurance available to individuals and small groups on the same terms and conditions as those currently offered to employees of many large corporations under ERISA. Insurance companies that offer federally certified products would be required to meet financial structure and solvency requirements and would no longer be exempt from federal antitrust statutes under the McCarran-Ferguson Act. States would continue to supervise day-to-day market conduct.

The federal market would operate alongside existing state-regulated insurance markets, allowing individuals and employers to choose between state and federally regulated plans. The ability to choose between the two markets would serve as a check on the imposition of regulation that is ultimately not in consumers' interests. If one level of government imposes undesirable rules in one market, consumers will have the opportunity to vote with their feet for insurance plans in the other.

The reform will also create several ancillary benefits. First, it will increase the portability of health insurance. Families that currently purchase insurance in the individual or small-group market in one state often must drop that coverage and find new insurance when moving to another state. At a minimum, this exposes the family to unnecessary financial risks. With nationwide, competitively priced insurance plans available, the potential loss of insurance will no longer be a barrier to relocation.

Second, the policy change will create a more level playing field between families that must obtain insurance in the non-group market and those who work for large employers whose plans are exempt from costly state regulations. And the reduction in costs will lead to a decline in the uninsured.

The main concern about this proposal is that it will lead to even more regulation than occurs under state law. By increasing the scope of federal control, Congress would be capable of imposing broad regulations across the entire U.S. market with a single vote. If individual states retained jurisdiction, then separate actions by fifty state legislatures would be required to achieve the same regulatory outcome.

Indeed, this is precisely what has happened with the enactment in 2010 of the PPACA. The policy choice we now face is to (1) repeal the act entirely, return to the highly inefficient system of state regulation, and hope that future Congresses will refrain from re-regulating insurance markets; or (2) replace the act with rules that will allow market incentives to demonstrate their effectiveness. We propose the latter choice. We would eliminate community rating, most minimum benefit regulations, and minimum medical loss ratios, all of which are now the law of the land.

A second policy alternative is to allow individuals and small groups to shop across state lines for insurance.[41] Initially, this policy would make available insurance plans that are free of mandates and regulations imposed by the state in which the individual resides, but which are not imposed in other states. Over time, this policy would create competition among states to establish a regulatory environment that allows for a more attractive and less costly set of insurance options.

Although allowing interstate shopping can help instigate a national market in insurance, it has two potential drawbacks, to the extent that it essentially assigns all regulatory responsibility to the insurer's state. This could be problematic if it encourages states to choose regulatory regimes that externalize costs onto insured individuals who live elsewhere. In addition, assigning all responsibility to the insurer's state will be inevitably resisted by some state insurance regulators and consumer groups. This resistance will result in lawsuits in state courts and/or congressional action, and the consequent uncertainty will inhibit firms from participating in the new market. For these reasons, some formal compromise apportionment of regulatory responsibility among the insurer's state, the insured's state, and the federal government is necessary; the apportionment we suggest is only one among many feasible policy options.

Subsidize Insurance for the Chronically Ill. As many thoughtful analysts have recognized, one of health policy's most vexing problems is providing affordable health insurance for chronically ill persons who, through no fault of their own, have predictably high medical expenses year after year and lack sufficient resources to finance them. Competitive markets for insurance, which provide good protection for unforeseen major medical expenses, do not work well for persistently high-cost patients.

Other responses to this problem have fared poorly. One response has been community rating, which has the adverse unintended consequences previously described. The other response has been high-risk pools. In principle, high-risk pools allow individuals who have been denied coverage or charged a high premium due to their health status to obtain subsidized insurance. In 1999, although twenty-eight states operated high-risk pools, they covered a total of only 105,000 individuals.[42] The authors of this study concluded that the small size of pool enrollment is due to several factors, including high costs, limited benefits, limited outreach to prospective members, and, in some cases, explicitly capped enrollment.

We propose making persons suffering from chronic illnesses eligible for a public subsidy to purchase insurance in the nationwide private insurance market. In order to be eligible for the subsidy, chronically ill persons would be required to have been covered by insurance in the past and have insufficient resources to pay for their own coverage. This proposal expands on the temporary "reinsurance" fund created by the PPACA.

The subsidy would provide partial coverage to an eligible person free of charge that would begin to cover health care expenses when they exceeded a specified multiple of that person's area-average expenses. The partial insurance could only be used with a basic wrap-around policy purchased from an insurer in the federal market. The subsidy could be implemented through a uniform federal program or through block grants to the states.

This subsidy would preserve coverage for the chronically ill at a lower cost than its alternatives, and without the unintended consequences and market distortions created by them. One alternative, for example, seeks to socialize the costs of all high-cost patients. Such socialization helps the chronically ill, but it also subsidizes the catastrophically ill—those with unexpectedly high costs that will not persist, such as individuals injured in auto accidents. Private insurance markets, however, work well at financing the care of the catastrophically ill; adverse selection arises only when a patient's (high) expenditures are predictable in advance.

The extra cost of this alternative could be substantial. According to a 2003 study based on the Medical Expenditures Panel Survey, a large fraction of individuals who have high costs in one year do not have them in subsequent years.[43] The top 1 percent of users of health care services in 1996 accounted for 27.9 percent of all health care expenditures, the top 5 percent for 56 percent, and the top 10 percent for

69.8 percent.[44] However, only 13.7 percent of the top 1 percent of 1996 spenders were in the top 1 percent of 1997 spenders; approximately half of the top 1 percent of 1996 spenders remained in the top 10 percent.

In addition, a subsidy for the chronically ill could result in significantly lower insurance premiums for chronically ill persons who do not qualify for our proposed program. In theory, a subsidy to high-cost individuals, by reducing the range of hidden information in insurance markets, will dampen insurers' incentives to protect themselves against adverse selection. As incentives to protect against adverse selection decline, pooling increases, which would lead to increased insurance coverage of even *unsubsidized* high-cost individuals.[45]

In a recent paper that examines the impact of the 1973 extension of Medicare to the disabled, we find strong evidence of this important spillover benefit.[46] The extension had the effect of removing high-cost persons from the broader pool of privately insured persons. The greater the number of disabled persons Medicare removed from a state's private insurance pool, the greater the increase in private health insurance coverage among similar high-cost persons. Thus, the expansion of Medicare not only increased coverage among the targeted population of the disabled, but also among people who were similarly situated but less seriously impaired, suggesting the potential usefulness of subsidies to high-cost individuals in promoting insurance coverage generally.

These two reforms leave open the issue of what to do about individuals who have had continuous insurance coverage, develop a serious illness or injury through no fault of their own, and are confronted with higher insurance premiums when they seek to renew. Concerns about such individuals have driven much of the debate over insurance regulation, motivating such reforms as community rating and bans on insurance denial due to pre-existing conditions.

Yet, despite the intensity of these concerns, the problem's scope and magnitude are not known. In our review of the literature, we were unable to find any study that documented the number of people exposed to "re-underwriting" risk or the amount of premium increases that they faced. Without this information, the benefits and costs of competing regulatory solutions cannot be assessed.

What we do know suggests that the problem is limited. The Health Insurance Portability and Accountability Act (HIPAA) protects all individuals with employer-sponsored coverage from re-underwriting risk by mandating that their coverage be "guaranteed renewable" and prohibiting differential pricing within a firm. From the work of Patel and Pauly (2002), we also know that forty-seven states and the District of Columbia prohibit rate increases upon renewal in the individual insurance market based on changes in health. Although individuals transitioning from employer-sponsored to individual insurance are not guaranteed complete protection against premium increases, HIPAA does require insurers to offer "HIPAA Conversion" policies in the individual market without pre-existing condition exclusions to anyone with sufficient creditable employer-sponsored coverage; forty-six states regulate these policies' premiums.[47] And, although there is no definitive evidence on the effectiveness of state guaranteedrenewability rules, work by Bradley Herring and Mark Pauly suggests that enforcing this regulation should not be difficult if consumers truly want guaranteed-renewable coverage.[48]

REDESIGN MEDICARE AND MEDICAID

Medicare. Although Medicare began in 1965 as a one-size-fits-all, fee-for-service insurance program, changes to it since then have steadily increased the role of beneficiary choice and private health plans.[49] In 1982, the Tax Equity and Fiscal Responsibility Act (TEFRA) made it easier and more attractive for private health maintenance organizations to contract with Medicare. In 1997, the Balanced Budget Act (BBA) expanded the types of private organizations that could contract with the program, formally creating Medicare Part C, also known as "Medicare+Choice." By 2000, 17 percent of Medicare beneficiaries had enrolled in private plans through this part of the program.[50]

This experience was important in the passage of the Medicare Prescription Drug, Improvement, and Modernization Act of 2003, which renamed the Medicare+Choice program "Medicare Advantage" and created Medicare Part D, a voluntary outpatient prescription drug benefit that was entirely administered by private plans. By all accounts, Medicare Part D has been highly successful. A 2010 survey conducted by the Healthcare Leadership Council found very high levels of beneficiary satisfaction with Part D.[51] According to the Office of the Actuary at the Centers for Medicare and Medicaid Services, Part D is now forecast to cost $261 billion less than was initially predicted for the 2004–2013 period—a 41 percent savings.[52] Research by Mark Duggan and Fiona

Scott Morton suggests that this cost saving was due, at least in part, to effective negotiations by the plans over prescription drug prices.[53]

We propose taking Medicare the next step and begin transforming it into the Part D model. We would give beneficiaries a risk-adjusted payment with which to purchase coverage in a regulated marketplace. However, the current rules that limit Medicare Advantage plans' freedom to offer benefits that differ from traditional fee-for-service Medicare must be changed. We propose that the current rules be relaxed to allow plans to offer choices that involve significantly more cost-sharing and/or other controls on the use of services.

This change will enable beneficiaries to become more engaged in their health care decisions. It will also facilitate more innovative payment systems for physician and hospital services. These changes are two keys to modernizing the Medicare program and bringing its costs under control.

Medicaid. Medicaid was created in 1965 to provide matching funds for states to care for the medically indigent.[54] State participation in the program was (and still is) voluntary. Originally, all persons eligible for Aid to Families with Dependent Children (AFDC) were automatically eligible for Medicaid, but states were allowed to determine their own eligibility standards for AFDC. Over time, however, federal legislation has reduced states' discretion over Medicaid eligibility standards. In 1984, for example, states were required to extend coverage to low-income women and children in two-parent families. By 1990, federal law required states to cover all low-income pregnant women and children under age six. The PPACA effectively eliminated states' discretion over eligibility by mandating coverage of all individuals under age sixty-five with income up to 133 percent of the federal poverty level beginning in 2014.

Along these lines, the benefits that states must cover have also been specified in federal statutes and regulations, and have included a wide range of non-acute, acute, and long-term care services and supplies. Just as with eligibility, the PPACA has also essentially eliminated states' discretion over what benefits must be covered; among other things, PPACA mandates that states' Medicaid programs cover all "essential health benefits."[55]

One reason why the federal government has expanded the scope of Medicaid so dramatically is that it's paying for only slightly more than half of the cost of the program—in 2010, 56.4 percent.[56] Until recently, when the sheer magnitude of the program grew so large that it threatened states' solvency, states have also had an incentive to expand Medicaid, for the same reason.

This program design is inherently flawed. Under this shared financing arrangement, each level of government bears only a portion of the cost of any program expansion and receives only a portion of any savings from programmatic reductions. We propose to transform Medicaid into a block grant to the states. Although the appropriate size of Medicaid is a matter for political debate, the only way to reach a considered decision in a federal system is for the full cost of the program to be borne by the entity that determines the program's scope. The block grant approach, by properly aligning federal and state incentives, has been highly successful in bringing under control federal and state cash welfare costs without creating hardship for recipients.

Expand Provision of Health Information

If health care markets are to work effectively and consumers are to make wise choices about their care, they need more access to better information about quality and cost. We focus on two approaches to improving the provision of health information: report cards and clinical practice guidelines.

Report cards collect and disseminate data on the quality of doctors, hospitals, nursing homes, and health plans. Clinical practice guidelines specify the right kind of treatment for a specific illness, set of symptoms, or type of patient. Both the public and private sectors have developed extensive sets of report cards and clinical practice guidelines. Yet surveys of health-services research provide at best equivocal evidence of the effectiveness of these vehicles for improving consumer information.[57]

We propose two initiatives to enhance the effectiveness of report cards and clinical practice guidelines. First, we propose supporting a privately produced portfolio of different types of report cards with public funds and publicly collected data. As with many grants through the U.S. Department of Health and Human Services (HHS) and the National Institutes of Health (NIH), these grants could be accompanied by permission to use health-insurance claims and mortality data from individual states or the Medicare and Medicaid programs. Indeed, HHS and NIH already provide such confidential data to researchers for this and similar purposes. In particular, we would emphasize research that seeks to measure the effects on patient decision-making of different types of report cards. We would also emphasize research that seeks to measure the extent to which compensating doctors, hospitals, and insurers on the basis of report cards enhances their utility to consumers.

Second, we propose that HHS improve its efforts to encourage use of generally recommended treatments through the development and dissemination of guidelines, keeping in mind that while guidelines can help practicing physicians make use of the most recent scientific research, blind adherence to them runs the risk of one-size-fits-all medicine.

The Surgeon General can help to make guidelines easier for physicians and patients to use. More accessible guidelines not only serve to inform physicians of best practices, they also alert patients to the onset of illness and encourage them to become more involved in their health care decisions. We propose that the Surgeon General, in consultation with HHS, physician organizations, state health departments, and insurers, identify the most costly and prevalent illnesses whose generally accepted best practices are not universally followed, post these illnesses with their respective guidelines on the Internet, and undertake a public-service campaign to increase patient and physician compliance.

Control Anticompetitive Behavior

As with the functioning of insurance markets, we also have many of the tools necessary to control private anticompetitive behavior. American antitrust laws have protected consumers and promoted free markets that have made the U.S.

economy the strongest in the world. We have already proposed that the exemption from antitrust laws for insurers
under the McCarran-Ferguson Act be sharply limited. In
addition, public policy can take further steps to ensure competitive health care markets. Three practices should receive
top priority from the antitrust enforcement agencies.

First, we propose aggressive investigation of mergers
among hospitals that lead to very high concentrations of
market power. Recent research shows that such concentrations both raise costs and reduce quality.[58] For Medicare beneficiaries suffering from heart attack, the costs of care in the
most competitive areas were approximately 8 percent lower
than those in the least competitive areas, and mortality after
one year approximately 4 percent lower.[59] When doctors
and their patients lack choices, hospitals lose the incentive
to provide effective and efficient care.

Second, we propose to limit strictly the ability of doctors
and hospitals to boycott patients and their health plans in order
to obtain anticompetitive concessions on prices and quality.
Many believe that allowing doctors and hospitals the latitude
to join together against health plans will only affect the health
plans' profits, not costs for consumers. They are mistaken.
Increases in prices and health care costs translate into higher
premiums for firms and workers, rising rates of uninsurance,
and higher costs for the Medicare and Medicaid programs.

Third, we propose exploration of the existence and
potential effects of barriers to the entry into the field of new
physicians and specialists. The Accreditation Council for
Graduate Medical Education (ACGME), a private organiza-
tion controlled by physicians and hospitals, exercises vir-

tually complete control in every specialty over the number of residency programs and the number of residents in each program—and therefore over the flow of new physicians.[60] An agreement by industry participants to limit entry of new competitors is generally considered a violation of the antitrust laws: why should health care be different? Graduate medical education must be subject to rigorous quality controls, but this goal can be accomplished without the anticompetitive effects of the ACGME's current approach.

Reform the Malpractice System

Research on medical malpractice litigation by both academics and government agencies is clear: The broken litigation system leads to fewer choices for patients and to higher costs because of "defensive medicine." As a first step to reforming the malpractice system, we propose reasonable, national caps on noneconomic damages in medical malpractice lawsuits. According to the Medical Liability Monitor, doctors in Nevada, Pennsylvania, Mississippi, North Carolina, Virginia, Florida, and Ohio—all states without reasonable limits on noneconomic damages in 2001—had annual increases in their malpractice premiums from 2001–02 of between 40 and 113 percent.[61]

Evidence that these increases have led to decreases in physician availability, particularly among specialists, is persuasive. Two recent studies report that states adopting reforms that directly reduce liability, such as caps on noneconomic damages, experienced significantly greater growth in physicians per capita over the 1980s and 1990s than states without such caps.[62]

In addition to fewer choices, malpractice pressure leads to higher health care costs beyond its direct impact on malpractice insurance. Not only do doctors and hospitals pass on the direct costs of increased malpractice premiums, they provide more expensive and relatively unproductive medical treatments out of fear of litigation. The additional cost of defensive medicine attributable to the medical liability system is estimated to range from 3 to 7 percent (box 6).[63]

Three alternative reforms to the tort system also hold significant promise. First, systems of error-reporting, analysis, and feedback—which are central to efforts to reduce medical errors—should be protected from liability. The most important impediment to the creation and success of these systems is the discoverability of their data by potential plaintiffs in medical malpractice lawsuits. States differ in the extent to which they protect analyses of medical errors by hospitals, physician groups, and insurers from lawsuits. Such analyses are generally discoverable by plaintiffs, unless the analysis falls under a state's specific statutory exception.[64] However, even states with these statutory exceptions do not generally protect information that is shared across organizations.

Consistent with findings of the Institute of Medicine[65] and many bills that have been introduced in Congress, we propose to limit the discoverability in a legal proceeding of data on adverse events collected for purposes of quality improvement. Such legal protection will encourage health care organizations to develop policies to collect and analyze

BOX 6
The Costs of Defensive Medicine

How costly is defensive medicine, and how effective are legal reforms at reducing its prevalence? To investigate this question, Daniel Kessler and Mark McClellan analyzed longitudinal data on essentially all elderly Medicare beneficiaries hospitalized with serious cardiac illness from 1984 to 1994, matched with information on the medical malpractice liability reforms in effect in the state in which each patient was treated.[66] They modeled the effect of reforms on total hospital expenditures on the patient in the year after the onset of illness and on important patient outcomes, and they estimated the effect of reforms on a serious adverse outcome that is common in our study population: mortality within one year of occurrence of the cardiac illness. They also estimated the effect of reforms on two other common adverse outcomes related to a patient's quality of life—whether the patient experienced a subsequent heart attack or heart failure requiring hospitalization in the year following the initial illness. They compared trends in treatments, costs, and outcomes for patients from states reforming their liability system to patients from non-reforming states, holding constant patient background characteristics, state of residence and year, and the legal and political characteristics of states.

Kessler's and McClellan's analysis indicated that reforms that directly limited liability—such as caps on damages—reduced hospital expenditures by 3–7 percent, depending on the type of patient and the market environment. In contrast, reforms that limited liability only indirectly were not associated with any substantial expenditure effects. Neither type of reform led to any consequential differences in mortality or the occurrence of serious complications. Thus, treatment of elderly patients with heart disease does involve defensive medical practices, and limited reductions in liability can reduce this costly behavior.

(continued on following page)

> (Box 6 *continued*)
>
> Recent work has updated these findings and extended them to broader groups of individuals. Baicker, Fisher, and Chandra (2007) report that states in the top quartile of malpractice payments per physician have total Medicare spending that is 4.2 percent higher than states in the bottom quartile of malpractice payments per physician. Hellinger and Encinosa (2006) report that states that directly limit liability have 3–4 percent lower health spending overall than states that do not.

information about medical errors and encourage health care workers to report mistakes. Passing such legislation would be an important step toward reducing medical errors.

Second, patients and providers should be given more freedom to experiment with alternatives to the courts. In binding alternative dispute resolution (ADR), patients and providers voluntarily submit disputes to an arbitrator who resolves the case in a binding decision. According to its proponents, ADR compensates victims faster, more fairly, and with lower transaction costs. ADR also can enhance the incentives for doctors and hospitals to take more appropriate precautions against medical errors, by replacing the current compensation lottery with a more consistent decision-making process.[67]

Yet ADR is surprisingly uncommon. Its proponents argue that state laws and judicial decisions that make ADR agreements impossible to enforce leave arbitrators powerless. According to this reasoning, few agree to ADR because its decisions do not mean much. Opponents of ADR argue that bias in favor of defendants, or at least the perception of bias, is responsible for its unpopularity. According to this reasoning, patients are wary of ADR because arbitrators are more likely to develop ties to the provider organizations that pay for their services than to individual plaintiffs.

Before we give up on ADR, we need to reform public policy to give it a chance. To give everyone more confidence in ADR, legal and regulatory reform should ensure that its decisions are both enforceable and impartial.

Third, we propose to study adoption of a guidelines-based rule for adjudicating physician negligence in malpractice claims. Under the common law of most states, physician negligence is an issue of fact for the jury, informed by expert testimony. Under a guidelines-based system, compliance with a guideline could be allowed as a defense to malpractice; failure to comply with a guideline, without a patient's written permission, could be allowed as evidence of malpractice. Although guidelines are an obvious source of information about the negligence of a given treatment decision in a medical malpractice case, courts generally bar them from being admitted as evidence under the hearsay rule, which prohibits the introduction of out-of-court statements as evidence. Guidelines are sometimes admitted under the "learned treatise" exception to the hearsay rule. Under most states' common law, no one set of guidelines necessarily trumps any other, and they carry no more weight than any other form of expert testimony.[68] Thus, adoption of a guidelines-based system would require legislative action.

Several states have already experimented with legal reforms that make evidence of compliance with guidelines statutorily admissible by defendants as an affirmative defense to malpractice. For example, Florida and Maine passed laws creating demonstration projects in the 1990s that allowed physicians to opt into a guidelines-based malpractice system.[69] Because there are many contexts in which medical care is widely known to deviate from "best practices," expanding the role of guidelines has the potential to improve the quality of care further.

Study the Tax Preference for Nonprofits

Finally, we propose that the Departments of Treasury and HHS study whether current government policy governing the tax exemption for not-for-profit health care institutions is in the public interest. First, the empirical evidence about the exemption's effectiveness as a vehicle for promoting care for the poor is equivocal at best (see box 7). Second, to the extent that our proposed policy package increases insurance-coverage rates, tax subsidies for uncompensated care become less necessary. Third, the tax exemption protects nonprofit institutions from competition from for-profit institutions, thereby lessening the competitive pressures to make nonprofits as efficient as possible. Finally, the revenue gained from removing the tax exemption for nonprofits could be used to finance other improvements in health care coverage and treatment. One study calculated the revenue cost of the tax subsidy provided to nonprofit hospitals and found that in 1994–95, it amounted to $9.21 billion in 2002 dollars, including an exemption from income taxes of $5.43 bil-

BOX 7

The Consequences of For-Profit versus Nonprofit Ownership of Hospitals

Economists and health-policy scholars have long been interested in three potential consequences of for-profit versus nonprofit ownership of hospitals: the effect of ownership on the magnitude of benefits supplied to the community, the effect on productive efficiency, and the effect on tax revenues.

Most studies have found essentially no difference in the community benefits provided by for-profit versus nonprofit hospitals, where community benefits are defined to include uncompensated care and the provision of unprofitable or non-reimbursable services.[70] Indeed, some studies find that non-profits actually treat fewer indigent patients than for-profits.[71] There is some evidence that public hospitals that convert to for-profit status reduce the amount of uncompensated care they supply. However, public hospitals that convert supply much lower levels of uncompensated care before their conversion than public hospitals that do not convert.[72]

Evidence on the prices and/or costs of for-profit versus nonprofit hospitals is slightly more mixed. Some older studies find that for-profits have higher prices and/or costs, but more recent work suggests that these differences have shrunk or even reversed themselves.[73] There is also evidence that the presence of for-profits in an area leads to more efficient production of hospital services—even by nonprofits.[74]

lion, an exemption from property taxes of $2.01 billion, tax deductibility of donor contributions of $1.34 billion, and tax-exemption of interest paid on debt of $0.43 billion.[75]

CHAPTER 3

Impacts of Proposals on Health Care Spending, the Uninsured, the Federal Budget, and the Distribution of Tax Burdens

The U.S. health care system remains the finest in the world, leading in innovation and quality of care. At the same time, increasing failures in the workings of markets for health insurance and health care have fostered concerns that the system is too costly for all Americans and unavailable to some. The combination of third-party payment for most health care, weak incentives for consumers and producers, and a growing presence of government in health care financing spells trouble, both in terms of value and access today and stifled innovation in the future. The alternative is to alter incentives for consumers and providers in private health care markets.

We have proposed policy changes to empower consumers and improve competition and choice in health care markets. These changes are incremental—they can be implemented in most cases with simple modifications of existing law—but they set forth a powerful new policy direction by

promoting true health insurance, making consumers better
informed purchasers of health care, and enhancing competition in health insurance and health care markets. The
changes share a common goal—improving the ability of
private markets to insure and provide health care—thereby
benefiting Americans today through lower costs and greater
choice, and Americans in the future by providing the best
incentives for capturing the innovative possibilities in health
care in this century.

The steps we have outlined offer two significant potential
gains: a reduction in the resources spent on relatively unproductive care and a reduction in the number of uninsured.

Effects of Reforms on Health Care Spending

In this section, we summarize the effects of four of our policy
reforms on health care spending: tax deductibility, the tax
credit, insurance-market reforms, and malpractice reforms.
(These effects are listed in box 8.) In each case, we use estimates of the magnitude of behavioral responses from existing academic studies. A more complete description of these
behavioral responses and how they were used to obtain estimated impacts is provided in the appendices. We assume
that health care subsidies for the chronically ill will have no
impact on health spending and will primarily shift health
care expenditures from inefficient financing through health-
insurance regulation to direct subsidies.

Our estimates are based on data that reflect current
health care market conditions. The enactment of the Patient

BOX 8
Impact of Proposals on Health Care Spending, 2010

	Percent Change	Absolute Change ($ billion)
Tax Deductibility	–6.2	–63
Tax Credit	+0.7	+7
Insurance-Market Reforms	–1.0	–10
Medical Malpractice Reform	–1.7	–18
Total	**–8.2**	**–84**

Source: Authors' calculations.

Protection and Affordable Care Act of 2010 will significantly alter the health care landscape beginning in 2014. But, the impact of its provisions is not known with sufficient precision to incorporate its effects formally into our analysis. Our discussion includes a less formal treatment in areas where it is most important.

TAX DEDUCTIBILITY

We begin with the impact of tax deductibility. Allowing out-of-pocket health care spending to be tax-deductible has two opposing effects on health care spending. First, expanding deductibility lowers the overall price of health care relative to other goods and services and, thereby, increases spending. Second, expanding deductibility raises the price of purchasing health care through insurance relative to purchasing such care out of pocket. The second effect induces people to shift to health plans with higher deductibles and coinsurance rates which, in turn, lowers spending.

Our key result is that the expenditure-reducing effect of full deductibility is greater in magnitude than the expenditure-increasing effect. We are not the first researchers to recognize this possibility.[1] This result is important for two reasons. First, it implies that full deductibility is an effective policy to address rising health care costs. Second, it has important implications for the policy's impact on the federal budget. Reductions in health care expenditures that come from removing the tax-favored status of health insurance are not a loss to the economy; that is, GDP will not decline by the reduction in health care spending. The tax-free resources no longer used for health care consumption will be channeled to other, taxable, economic activities. The resulting increase in tax revenues will offset a significant amount of the loss from making out-of-pocket health care expenditures tax-deductible.

We calculate the total effect of deductibility in two steps. First, we calculate the extent to which full deductibility would reduce the after-tax price of out-of-pocket spending. Across all taxpayers, we estimate that this price would decline by about 15 percent. Second, we calculate the responsiveness of total health expenditures to a decrease in this price. Based on estimates from the literature, we calculate that each 1 percent decrease in the after-tax price of out-of-pocket expenditures would reduce total health expenditures (on insurance and out-of-pocket) by 0.41 percent (see Appendix A). Hence, full deductibility would reduce health care spending by 6.2 percent (= 0.41 × 15 percent).

These savings of approximately 6 percent in private health spending would translate into modestly higher coinsurance rates and dramatically lower expenditures on health insurance. A 6.2 percent reduction amounts to a $63 billion reduction in aggregate U.S. private health care spending in 2010. In Appendix D, we show that if this reduction were achieved entirely through a rise in coinsurance rates, the typical coinsurance rate would rise from 25 to 33 percent.

TAX CREDIT

Implementation of the health care tax credit would raise overall health care spending as each newly insured recipient increased his use of health care services. We estimate that the tax credit would increase the number of insured individuals by 6 million. If each newly insured person increased his spending by 50 percent, aggregate U.S. health care spending would rise by about $7 billion per year in 2010. Thus, increases in health care spending due to the tax credit would offset the $63 billion decline due to deductibility, but only by a small amount (Appendix A).

INSURANCE-MARKET REFORM

In our previous discussion of insurance-market reforms, we noted that the Congressional Budget Office had estimated that eliminating state benefits mandates alone would reduce the cost of a typical insurance plan by 5 percent and possibly as much as 15 percent.[2] Similarly, eliminating any-willing-provider laws would reduce the cost of insurance by nearly 2 percent.[3]

Based upon the lower end of the range of estimates by the Congressional Budget Office, our proposed insurance reforms would reduce the cost of insurance by 7 percent. Because individuals would respond to lower insurance costs by increasing their insured expenditures, we estimate that insurance-market reforms would reduce health care spending by only 1 percent, or $10 billion per year (Appendix A).

MALPRACTICE REFORM

In our previous discussion of malpractice reforms, we reported that the additional cost of defensive medicine attributable to the medical liability system is estimated to be in the range of 3–7 percent. We assume that limits on noneconomic damages would reduce the overall cost of care by the lower end of this range, 3 percent. Allowing for individuals to respond to this reduction by increasing their purchases of care would reduce the impact to 1.7 percent, or $17 billion per year (Appendix A).

SUMMARY AND DISCUSSION

Taken together, the four proposals discussed here would reduce total health care spending by 8.2 percent, or $84 billion per year.

As we noted earlier, PPACA is expected to increase health care spending dramatically starting in 2014. If its provisions become effective, particularly the employer and individual mandates that everyone must have health insurance, our proposals to reduce costs become more important. The dollar amount of health care spending reductions from our proposals should rise in proportion to increases in health care costs from the 2010 legislation.

The most common criticisms of our proposals are of two types: that our expenditure saving depends upon unrealistic estimates of the responsiveness of health spending to copayment rates; and that higher copayment rates will not have much effect on the bulk of medical expenditures, which are incurred by the chronically or terminally ill. In our view, neither of these criticisms is strong.

First, calculations of the overall impact of our policies on spending are not particularly sensitive to the magnitude of the response of health spending to its effective price. Even if individuals' behavioral response is half as great as we assume it is, the total effect of our package on health spending would be 8.7 percent—greater than the estimate we use of 8.2 percent. The composition of savings would shift from being primarily due to deductibility to being due about equally to deductibility, insurance-market reform, and malpractice reform (see Appendix A for details); but the bottom-line total would be roughly the same.

Second, health insurance based on health savings accounts combined with a catastrophic plan can, in practice, subject most expenditures to the discipline of "spending your own money." Two common arguments against this proposition—the high persistence of expenditures and the high cost of end-of-life care—are far weaker than they are commonly believed to be. Matthew Eichner, Mark McClellan, and David Wise analyzed the health-insurance claims of a large Fortune 500 manufacturing company from 1989 to 1991.[4]

They report that among employees ages forty-six to fifty-five
with health expenditures of at least $5,000 in 1989 (roughly
the top decile of spenders), only 28.6 percent had expenditures of at least $5,000 in 1990.[5] Alan Monheit's analysis of
the data from the Medical Expenditure Panel Survey finds
persistence that is somewhat greater, although not substantially so.[6] Among individuals in the top decile of spenders in
1996, 37.9 percent remained in the top decile in 1997.[7]

Although the cost of end-of-life care is not trivial, the
share of Medicare expenditures incurred in the last year of
life has remained roughly constant over the past twenty years
at one-quarter of the total.[8] Thus, even if higher deductibles
and copayments could not affect the cost of care at the end
of life, they could still affect three-quarters of the level—and
growth—in expenditures. In addition, there is evidence that
the same incentives that affect the cost of care of chronically
ill survivors also affect the care of chronically ill decedents.
It is generally not possible to predict individual patient
mortality with sufficient specificity to influence medical
decision-making, even with detailed clinical records. The
characteristics of Medicare decedents are similar to those of
high-cost survivors.[9]

Effects of Reforms on the Number of Uninsured

We have developed a four-pronged policy to reduce the number of uninsured persons: full above-the-line tax deductibility of both insurance premiums and out-of-pocket expenses;
tax credits; and malpractice and insurance-market reforms

to make health insurance more affordable, more portable, and better tailored to individuals' needs.

TAX DEDUCTIBILITY

Full tax deductibility would decrease the price of insurance for a large number of uninsured persons. According to the National Institute for Health Care Management Foundation, nearly half of the uninsured (about 20 million) would benefit from tax deductibility; between 2 million and 6 million would be induced to purchase insurance (see Appendix B for details).

TAX CREDIT

The tax credit would further reduce the number of uninsured. According to data from the Medical Expenditure Panel Survey, one in every five non-elderly uninsured individuals is in a household earning less than the poverty threshold, and nearly half are in households earning 100–300 percent of the poverty threshold. How many of these 30 million persons would be induced to purchase health insurance as a consequence of the tax credit is subject to considerable empirical uncertainty. Using estimates from Mark Pauly and Bradley Herring, we estimate that between 3 million and 8 million individuals would do so (see Appendix B).

INSURANCE-MARKET AND MALPRACTICE REFORMS

Allowing insurance companies to sell policies free from state benefit-mandates and any-willing-provider laws on a nationwide basis would reduce costs by approximately 7 percent; malpractice reforms would produce a 3 percent reduction. In addition, our reforms would make insurance more portable and therefore more attractive, holding price constant. We estimate that the insurance-market and malpractice reforms would reduce the number of uninsured by between 2 million and 7 million individuals (see Appendix B).

SUMMARY AND DISCUSSION

Taken together, our proposed policy changes are projected to reduce the number of uninsured persons by 7 million to 21 million. The impact of these proposals on the ranks of uninsured, while substantial in their own right, might be even greater than these calculations suggest. For example, the more than 14 million uninsured Americans who are eligible for—but not enrolled in—government programs like Medicaid and/or SCHIP could also benefit from a more viable individual market, because Medicaid and SCHIP waivers can redirect existing (unused) funds into insurance vehicles to cover these individuals.

In addition, our policies are unlikely to increase the number of uninsured individuals by inducing employers to stop offering health insurance to their employees. Our policy of full deductibility retains a significant tax incentive for purchase of employer-provided insurance, so that any transition to a new mix of individual versus employer-sponsored insurance would be gradual. In particular, our proposal only allows the deduction of the cost of individual insurance from the income-tax base, not from the payroll-tax base. Expenditures on insurance purchased through an employer would, as under current law, still be excludable from both the income- and payroll-tax bases.

However, existing empirical evidence suggests that even if the after-tax prices of individual insurance and employer-provided insurance were fully equalized, employers' dropping of insurance would not be commonplace. Even in the absence of any tax preference, employers would only cease to offer insurance if their workers' demands for insurance were so different that the gains to low-demand workers from buying less insurance in the individual market outweighed the loss to all workers of the individual market's higher administrative costs. Research by Pauly, Percy, and Herring shows that this is unlikely to be the case. Under plausible assumptions about the extent of the differences in employees' demand for insurance at a typical firm, they report that the average benefit to an employee of opting out of his employer-provided insurance plan (in the absence of any tax preference) is approximately equal to the average cost, in terms of the increased administrative expenses, that he would face in the individual versus the group-insurance market.[10]

Our estimated reduction in the number of uninsured persons is from a current base of 46 million people.[11] The PPACA's employer and individual health insurance mandates and subsidies will, according to the CBO, reduce the number of uninsured persons by 15 million by 2017.[12] This estimate is well within the 7–21 million person reduction we estimate for our combined proposals. We have recommended that the PPACA's insurance mandates and subsidies be repealed. If they are repealed and our proposals are substituted in their place, we would expect no change in the number of uninsured persons.

Effects of Reforms on the Federal Budget

We now present the federal budget impact of our main policy reforms. For purposes of calculation, these include the four reforms mentioned above—tax deductibility, the tax credit, and insurance-market and malpractice reforms—plus health care subsidies for the chronically ill. We have not included the impact of our Medicare and Medicaid proposals in our formal estimates due to uncertainty about their magnitude. The calculations are based on 2010 data when possible, and inflated to 2010 terms if 2010 data were not available at the time of writing. Appendix D contains the details behind the calculations described below.

TAX DEDUCTIBILITY

Deductibility has two effects on revenues—a loss from making previously taxable spending deductible, and a gain from the shift away from previously deductible health spending. We do not account for any possible spillover effects from privately purchased health care to the Medicare or Medicaid programs.

The revenue *loss* consists of two components: the loss from allowing the above-the-line deduction of out-of-pocket spending and the loss from purchases on health insurance being deducted above the line that are currently not deducted or deductible. The revenue *gain* also consists of two components. Tax revenues rise because higher policy deductibles will translate into a shift in employees' compensation away from excludable health spending to taxable wages.[13] The government picks up both payroll and income taxes on the portion of the wage increase directed to non-health spending (first component), and payroll taxes on the portion directed to out-of-pocket health spending (second component).

To calculate the first component of the revenue loss, we multiply our estimate of the out-of-pocket-spending-weighted marginal tax rate, 0.14, by our estimate of the currently non-deducted out-of-pocket spending, $166 billion; this amount totals $23 billion. To calculate the second component of the revenue loss, we multiply 0.14 by our estimate of currently non-deducted (or non-deductible) health insurance spending, $86 billion; this totals $12 billion. The sum of these two components, $35 billion, is the gross revenue loss from the policy.

Tax deductibility will also lead to two revenue gains: one from a reduction in overall health spending and one from a shift in how medical care is purchased, away from insurance and toward out-of-pocket spending. To calculate the first gain, we multiply the reduction in overall spending, $63 billion, by the health-spending-weighted average marginal income tax rate plus the health-spending-weighted average payroll tax rate, 0.32; this amount totals $20 billion. To calculate the second gain, we multiply the increase in out-of-pocket spending, $63 billion, by the health-spending-weighted average payroll tax rate, 0.13; this amount totals $8 billion. The sum of these two components, $28 billion, is the gross revenue gain from the policy.

Combining the estimates of the revenue losses and gains from tax deductibility, we estimate its net impact to be a revenue loss of $7 billion.

TAX CREDIT

The revenue loss from the tax credit is the sum of two components—the cost from the use of the credit by currently insured individuals and the cost from its use by newly insured individuals. The credit's use by currently insured persons would cost the treasury $7 billion in annual revenues; its use by newly insured persons would cost another $6 billion (see Appendix D for details).

INSURANCE-MARKET AND MALPRACTICE REFORMS

We estimate that insurance-market and malpractice reforms would reduce overall health spending by 2.7 percent, or $28 billion. This transfer of health spending to other economic activities would generate a $7 billion increase in annual federal revenues.

SUBSIDY FOR THE CHRONICALLY ILL

The revenue loss from our proposal to provide federal subsidies for the chronically ill would depend upon three key parameters: the number of eligible people who take up the subsidy, the average health care costs per eligible person, and the generosity of the subsidy. We do not recommend a particular set of policy parameters at this juncture; instead, we offer an example for purposes of illustration.

In our example, we assume our proposed subsidy would cover approximately two-thirds more people than were covered by all state high-risk pools together, or 175,000 people.[14] This difference would amount to approximately 1 percent of the estimated number of people who would purchase insurance in the new federal market. (We base our estimate of the initial size of the federal market on the number of nonelderly people in 2008 with private health insurance not obtained through their employer or a relative's employer—17,889,000.)[15]

For purposes of this example, we further assume that the subsidy would cover 75 percent of the expenses of an eligible person in excess of $15,000. According to the Medical Expenditure Panel Survey, the average health spending of the top 1 percent of the distribution of individuals with employer-sponsored insurance was $81,700 in 2007.[16] If we assume that the level of spending for this group grew at the same rate as did overall spending on health services and supplies from 2007–2010, then the average cost per person of the subsidy would be $57,279 in 2010, and the annual cost of the subsidy would be $57,279 × 175,000, or about $10 billion.[17]

SUMMARY AND DISCUSSION

Box 9 summarizes the total impact of our proposed policy changes on the federal budget.

The budget impact is estimated by comparing our policies to federal and state policies that are currently in place. The Patient Protection and Affordable Care Act, as we have previously noted, provides generous subsidies for individuals to purchase government-approved health plans starting in 2014. These provisions will increase federal budget outlays by $75 billion in 2017, according to CBO.[18] We have proposed that the subsidies and the new entitlement be

repealed. Using the projected growth rate on spending on
health services and supplies from CMS from 2010–2017,
these savings total $49 billion in 2010 dollars. Thus, our
proposals, combined with repeal of these two PPACA provisions, will reduce the annual federal budget deficit by about
$26 billion.

The inclusion of our Medicare proposals would produce
even larger reductions in the annual federal budget deficits. Recall, we estimated that increasing Medicare copayments to their mid-1970s levels would reduce Medicare
Part B expenditures by 29 percent. According to Table 13.1
of the Historical Tables of the 2011 U.S. Budget, payments
by Medicare Part B are expected to be $282.9 billion in
2010.[19] Thus, savings from our Medicare reforms would total
$82 billion in 2010. Including these savings would bring

BOX 9
Impact of Proposed Policies on
Federal Revenues, 2010

	Annual Revenue Impact
Tax Deductibility	–$7 billion
Tax Credit	–$13 billion
Insurance-Market and Malpractice Reforms	$7 billion
Subsidy for the Chronically Ill	–$10 billion
Total	**–$23 billion**

Source: Authors' calculations.

the reduction in the annual federal budget deficit to over
$100 billion.

Distributional Impact

We compute two measures of the distributional impact of our
tax policies using data from the 2002 Medical Expenditure
Panel Survey. The first measure is the percentage reduction in each income group's taxes that results solely from
tax deductibility (see figure 3); the second measure is the
same reduction when the credit is included (see figure 4).
We estimate the distributional effects of the credit under the

FIGURE 3

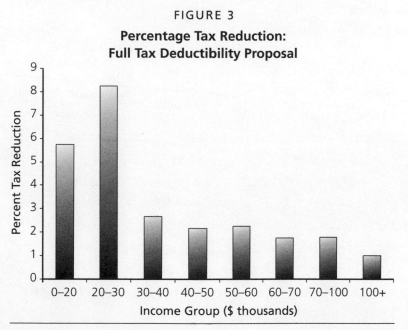

**Percentage Tax Reduction:
Full Tax Deductibility Proposal**

Source: Authors' calculations.

FIGURE 4

Percentage Tax Reduction:
Tax Deductibility and Tax Credit

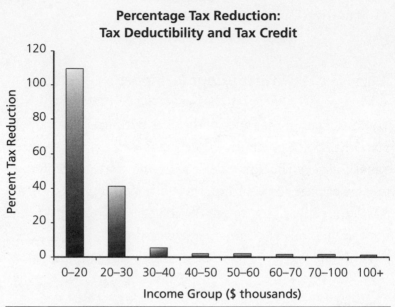

Income Group ($ thousands)

Source: Authors' calculations.

(very conservative) assumption that no individuals become newly insured due to the credit. Assuming no change in the income distribution, these measures are equal to the percentage change in tax burden as a share of income.

As figure 3 shows, the policy of making health care expenses tax-deductible is by itself progressive. Percentage tax reductions for low-income households are three to five times the same reductions for high-income households. For example, households earning less than $20,000 per year can expect a 5.7 percent reduction in their average tax rate, while households earning from $20,000 to $30,000 per year can expect an 8.3 percent reduction. This reduction comes about because our policy allows health expenses to be deducted "above the line"—that is, even by non-itemizing taxpayers. By comparison, households earning from $70,000 to $100,000 per year can expect only a 1.8 percent reduction in their average tax rate, and households earning more than $100,000 a 1 percent reduction.

As figure 4 shows, full deductibility combined with the tax credit is even more progressive. Households earning less than $20,000 per year can expect a 110 percent reduction in their average tax rate; households earning $20,000–$30,000 per year can expect a 41 percent reduction.

Conclusion

The U.S. health care system, the envy of the world in innovation, faces significant criticisms about cost, accessibility, and quality of care. While these criticisms are not without foundation, a more productive approach is to ask whether consumers of health care—and taxpayers in public financing—are obtaining the highest "value" for the resources devoted to health care. That is, are we getting what we should in return for the investments that we make, as individuals and a society, in our health care?

In our view, achieving this objective stands the greatest chance of success if health care markets function well. Market-based reform is neither a silver bullet nor a cure-all. Markets will not eliminate growth in health care costs—an inevitable product of technological change—or uninsurance. Markets will never solve the problem of how to finance care for the low-income chronically ill. But the power of markets to allocate resources efficiently—power evident in every other sector of the economy—is a critical part of the solution.

Yet markets cannot flourish without the appropriate institutional support for consumer incentives and choice, provider accountability, and competition. These needed features are held back in the United States in substantial measure by the unintended consequences of public policies in five areas. Any serious reform of the U.S. health care system must begin by changing these policies.

First, reform should increase individual involvement in health care decisions. The most important impediment to achieving this goal is the tax preference for employer-provided health insurance. Current tax policy generally allows people to deduct employer-provided health-insurance expenditures, but requires direct out-of-pocket medical spending to be made from after-tax income. This tax preference has given consumers the incentive to purchase health care through low-deductible, low-copayment insurance instead of out-of-pocket. This type of insurance has led to today's U.S. health care market in which cost unconsciousness and wasteful medical practices are the norm. The reason is, as the late Nobel laureate Milton Friedman once put it, "Nobody spends somebody else's money as wisely as he spends his own."[1]

The best way to reverse this trend would be to revoke the tax preference. Unfortunately, as the tax reform debates of the 1980s and the health reform debate of 2010 have shown, this solution appears politically infeasible. We propose a second-best solution: allow all Americans to deduct expenditures on health insurance and out-of-pocket expenses as long as they purchase at least catastrophic insurance. We show that under reasonable assumptions, expanding deductibility to out-of-pocket expenses will lead to a dramatic reduction in minimally productive health spending.

We are not the first researchers to recognize this possibility. Many economists and health-services researchers have recognized that expanding deductibility has two opposing effects on health care spending. First, it lowers the overall price of health care relative to other goods and services and, thereby, increases health care spending. Second, it raises the price of purchasing health care through insurance relative to out-of-pocket. The second effect induces people to shift to health plans with higher deductibles and coinsurance rates which, in turn, lowers health care spending. Because the base of out-of-pocket spending is so much smaller than that of insured spending, the net change in the overall price of health care from expanding deductibility is much smaller than the change in the relative price of out-of-pocket versus insured care. This fact leads the second effect to dominate the first and, in turn, leads to a net decrease in spending.

Expanding deductibility will have numerous other beneficial effects. Most notably, it will unambiguously reduce the rate of uninsurance. The most important cause of uninsurance is the high cost of health care. As we show, full deductibility significantly reduces the net cost of care for many of the uninsured, even those with moderate incomes. In addition, because the tax change allows the deductibility of out-of-pocket health care expenses only with the purchase of insurance, it creates a significant incentive for the currently uninsured to purchase insurance. Because it allows the deduction of the cost of individual insurance from the income-tax base but not from the payroll-tax base, the change retains a significant tax incentive for the purchase of employer-sponsored insurance as well. Expenditures on insurance purchased through an employer would, as under current law, still be excludable from both the income-tax and the payroll-tax base.

The tax change also enhances the fairness of the federal income-tax system. Under current law, individuals whose employers decline to offer them insurance are penalized because they must purchase it with after-tax income. Tax deductibility would promote tax simplicity by replacing the myriad of currently available special health care tax deductions discussed above with a single deduction equally applicable to all individuals. Finally, deductibility would increase the progressivity of the tax system. Although marginal tax rates are higher for higher-income people, the fact that lower-income people have higher (currently taxable) out-of-pocket spending more than compensates for this effect.

We combine the policy of full deductibility with other important changes to federal tax policy. To make it easier for individuals and families to save for expenses not covered by higher-deductible insurance, we propose allowing all individuals to contribute $1,800 per year ($3,700 maximum per household) to a health savings account, conditional on the purchase of insurance that covers at least catastrophic expenditures. As with current HSAs, balances may be spent on the health care of a relative, and those not spent on health care could be carried forward tax-free. Funds withdrawn for purposes other than health care would be subject to income tax. Recipients of health care tax credits (described below) could deposit funds in a health savings account if they wished. The purpose of these proposed changes is to make the current law governing HSAs less prescriptive and, thereby, to encourage greater use of HSAs. To improve the health care "safety net" for very-low-income households, we propose a refundable tax credit to offset their health expenses. While our proposal to make out-of-pocket medical expenses tax-deductible offers important benefits for many low- and middle-income working families, it does not help families that pay little or no income tax.

The second area in need of policy reform is the regulation of markets for health insurance. Like the tax preference, the unintended consequences of inefficient insurance regulation are to drive up costs and increase uninsurance. We propose that insurance companies that meet certain federal standards be permitted to offer plans on a nationwide basis free from costly state mandates, rules, and regulations. With this change, insurance would become available to individuals and small groups on the same terms and conditions as those currently available to employees of many large corporations who, because of a quirk in federal law, have been exempt from state insurance regulations for more than thirty years.

Given that approximately half of the insured U.S. population already obtains its insurance in what is effectively a federal market, this reform will not lead to radical or unpredictable changes in consumer protections. Federally certified health-insurance products would be required to meet all federal regulations that currently govern the provision of health insurance for large employers; there would be no rollback of existing federal health-insurance protections. Insurance companies that offer federally certified products would be required to meet financial structure and solvency requirements. In addition, states could continue to supervise day-to-day market conduct. Finally, insurance companies that offer federally certified products would no longer be exempt from federal antitrust statutes under the McCarran-Ferguson Act.

There are several benefits to creating a federally certified market for health insurance. Most importantly, this change will foster a more competitive, efficient, non-group health-insurance market that will enable individuals to obtain a greater variety of lower-cost alternatives. The lower cost will induce more people to buy insurance and, thereby, increase the size of risk pools—which will, in turn, further strengthen markets for insurance. In addition, a federal market will increase the portability of health insurance by making it easier for people to keep their insurance when they move across state lines.

Regulation of markets for insurance can be improved in another important way. To help competitive insurance markets provide affordable insurance for people with predictably high medical expenses year after year who lack sufficient resources to finance them, we propose making such people eligible for a subsidy to purchase insurance in the new nationwide market. A public-private partnership between the federal government and insurance companies would administer the subsidy. To be eligible, chronically ill persons would have to have been covered by insurance in the past and have insufficient resources to pay for their own coverage. Previous research has shown that states' current responses to the problem of the chronically ill—high-risk pools and insurance-rate regulation—have not addressed this important health policy problem. A targeted subsidy to those who are needy and suffering from insurance-market failure would provide a far more cost-effective solution.

The principles underlying the case for tax policy and insurance-market reform also have implications for government programs. To make individuals and health care providers more aware of the real resource costs of their decisions, the Medicare and Medicaid programs should have greater cost sharing. Of course, the extent of such cost sharing must take account of beneficiaries' income and health status to avoid preventing them from obtaining necessary care. Nonetheless, there is considerable room for change. The extent of cost-sharing in Medicare has fallen by approximately one-half since the 1970s. In particular, had Medicare's Part B (outpatient services) deductible kept pace with the increase in health spending, it would be approximately $700 today; instead, it is $162. At the very least, any future *additional* transfers to beneficiaries should come in the form of reductions in the growth in premiums, not reductions in copayments, which implies that the programs' cost-sharing going forward should increase at the rate of health spending growth.

Simply changing demand-side incentives in Medicare and Medicaid, however, is not enough. We must also fundamentally redesign the two programs. Medicare should be transformed into a program that gives beneficiaries a risk-adjusted payment with which to purchase coverage in a regulated marketplace. However, the current rules that limit Medicare Advantage plans' freedom to offer benefits that differ from traditional fee-for-service Medicare must be changed. In particular, plans must be allowed to offer choices that involve significantly more cost-sharing and/or other controls on the use of services. Medicaid should be transformed into a block grant to the states. The current structure of the program allows both federal and state governments to avoid bearing budgetary responsibility for their benefits and eligibility decisions and thereby creates powerful disincentives for cost control.

We also propose reforms in three additional areas: better provision of information to providers and consumers; an explicit public goal to control anticompetitive behavior by doctors, hospitals, and insurers; and reforms to the malpractice system to reduce wasteful treatment and medical errors. In each of these areas, research has indicated significant opportunities to achieve improvements in medical productivity that exceed the cost of the reforms.

Taken together, these changes harness the power of markets for health insurance and health care to deliver higher-value health care to Americans. They also allow markets to focus insurance and care arrangements more on individual needs. And better incentives promote consumers' ability to be cost- and value-conscious shoppers, as well as providers' accountability for quality and innovation in therapies, drugs, and medical devices. While the sweep of the reforms is radical, each change can be implemented as an incremental reform of the present U.S. health care system.

The time to implement these reforms is *now*. Failure to do so will exacerbate the problems of wasteful cost growth and a lack of insurance. It will also increase the pressure for more public intervention, with adverse consequences for innovation and flexibility. These problems have been *magnified* by the Patient Protection and Affordable Care Act of 2010, which put the crucial first step of cost containment and innovation in the back seat of a car driven by costly expansion of access within a system of flawed incentives. With this stark choice, health care is likely to be the center stage of domestic policy debates over the next decade.

APPENDIX A

Estimating the Impact of Policy Reforms on Health Care Spending

TAX DEDUCTIBILITY

We estimated the effect of extending deductibility to out-of-pocket spending on total spending in two steps. First, to determine how much deductibility would affect the after-tax price of out-of-pocket spending, we calculated a weighted-average marginal tax rate for all households, using each household's reported out-of-pocket expenses, including direct payments for health insurance by households without a self-employed person, as the weights. To do this, we used household-level data from the 2002 Medical Expenditure Panel Survey (MEPS) and inflated expenditures to 2004 levels using the Medical Consumer Price Index (MCPI).[1] We imputed a federal 2004 income-tax rate based upon the household's reported income and estimated tax deductions. We calculated a weighted-average marginal tax rate for all households, using each household's reported out-of-pocket expenses, including direct payments for health insurance by non-self-employed households, as the weights. We conclude that full deductibility would reduce the price of out-of-pocket health care relative to all other goods and services by 14 percent. Evaluated at the average after-tax price, this amounts to a 15 percent decrease ($= 0.14p_i / ((p_i^1 + (p_i - 0.14p_i)) / 2)$, where p_i is the before-tax price of insured expenditures).

Second, we calculated the effect on total health expenditures of a 1 percent increase in the after-tax price of out-of-pocket expenditures, as a function of the effect on total health expenditures of a 1 percent increase in the overall price of health care and the effect on total health expenditures of a 1 percent increase in the after-tax price of insured expenditures. This formula can be written:

$$e(t_o) \approx e(p) - e(t_i),$$

where $e(t_o)$ is the effect on total health expenditures of a 1 percent increase in the after-tax price of out-of-pocket expenditures; $e(p)$ is the effect on total health expenditures of a 1 percent increase in the overall price of health care; and $e(t_i)$ is the effect on total health expenditures of a 1 percent increase in the after-tax price of insured expenditures. (We prove this proposition in Appendix C.)

Both $e(p)$ and $e(t_i)$ are negative. Increases in the overall price of health care will lead to decreases in total expenditures; increases in the after-tax price of insured expenditures will lead to decreases in total expenditures as well. The effect on total expenditures of the after-tax price of insured expenditures consists of two components that work in the same direction. First, increasing the after-tax price of insured expenditures raises the overall price of health care relative to other goods and services and, thereby, lowers health care spending. Second, increasing the after-tax price of insured expenditures raises the price of purchasing health care through insurance relative to out of pocket. The second effect induces people to shift to health plans with higher deductibles and coinsurance rates which, in turn, lowers health care spending as well.

The sign of $e(t_o)$, then, depends on the relative magnitudes of $e(p)$ and $e(t_i)$. To assess the magnitude of $e(p)$, we look to two studies. Based on the RAND National Health Insurance Experiment, W. G. Manning and colleagues reported in 1987 that a 1 percent change in the coinsurance rate leads to a 0.2 percent decline in expenditures.[2] In more recent work, Eichner reports that a 1 percent change in the coinsurance rate leads to a 0.7 percent decline in expenditures (average for all employees 1990–92).[3] These are interpretable as arc elasticities $e(p)$ over coinsurance rates in the range of 25–50 percent.

We take two approaches to assessing the magnitude of $e(t_i)$. The first approach uses simulations based on theoretical models of insurance choice. To translate the results of these studies into an estimate of $e(t_i)$, we decompose $e(t_i)$ into two pieces, $e(c)$ and $e(c,t_i)$:

$$e(t_i) = e(c) \times e(c,t_i),$$

where $e(c)$ is the elasticity of spending with respect to the coinsurance rate and $e(c,t_i)$ is the elasticity of the coinsurance rate with respect to the tax preference for insured spending.

If demand curves are locally linear, then $e(p) = e(ap)$ for any positive constant a, so $e(c) = e(p)$, which implies:

$$e(t_i) = e(p) \times e(c,t_i).$$

Several studies have assessed the effect of the tax preference on coinsurance rates. These can be used to compute $e(c,t_i)$. Early simulations by Martin Feldstein and Bernard Friedman (1977) suggest that revoking the tax preference for employer-provided insurance would lead to a doubling in the coinsurance rate (from approximately 25 to 50 percent). This finding is consistent with an unpublished estimate by Charles Phelps (1986). More recent work leads to virtually the same conclusions. At conservative levels of consumer risk aversion and $e(p)$, simulations by Jack and Sheiner (1997, table 2) find that the tax preference for insurance has led optimal coinsurance rates to shrink from 33–67 percent to 20–30 percent. Assuming an average marginal (payroll plus income) tax rate of 30 percent, revocation leading to doubling of coinsurance rates from c to $2c$ implies an $e(c,t_i)$ in arc elasticity terms of 1.9, because:

$$\frac{\dfrac{2c-c}{[2c+c]} \Big/ 2}{\dfrac{1-(1-.3)}{[1+(1-.3)]} \Big/ 2} = 1.9.$$

At $e(p) = -0.45$ (the midpoint of the range of published estimates above), then, revoking the tax preference would lead to a decline in expenditures of 30 percent ($= -0.45 \times (50 - 25) / 37.5$). To translate this into an estimate of $e(t_i)$, we divide 30 percent by the percentage change in the after-tax price of insured expenditures that would result from revoking the tax preference. Assume that revoking the tax preference would raise the after-tax price of insured expenditures by about thirty percentage points. Evaluated at the average after-tax price, this amounts to a 35 percent increase (= $0.3p_i$ / ((p_i + (p_i − $0.3p_i$)) / 2), where p_i is the before-tax price of insured expenditures). Thus, a 1 percent increase in the after-tax price of insured expenditures translates into a 0.86 percent decrease in expenditures overall (= −0.30 / 0.35).

In a recent paper, we estimate $e(t_i)$ using the Medical Expenditure Panel Surveys from 1996–2005.[4] We use the fact that the Social Security program limits the annual amount of wage earnings that are subject to payroll taxation. Under the Social Security program, employers and employees each pay a 6.2 percent payroll tax on earnings below the maximum taxable wage (the "wage base"). The wage base is set by law and is automatically adjusted each year by the average growth in Social Security-covered wages. For workers who earn below the wage base, earnings are subject to payroll taxes while employer-sponsored health insurance premiums are not. This tax treatment of earnings, therefore, creates a 12.4 percent tax preference for insurance for these workers. For workers who earn above the wage base, neither earnings in excess of the threshold nor employer-sponsored health insurance premiums are subject to the payroll tax. For these workers there is, on the margin, no payroll tax preference for health insurance. By comparing health care spending of individuals in families with an employer-sponsored insurance policyholder who earns just below the maximum taxable wage to spending by individuals with a policyholder who earns just above this threshold, we can identify the impact of the tax preference on health care spending.

Comparing health care spending by workers below the threshold to those just above the threshold permits us to identify the impact of the tax preference. Using data from the full sample, we estimate $e(t_i)$ to be −0.74. If we exclude observations that are far from the discontinuity—which makes more plausible the identifying assumption that individuals on either side of the discontinuity are otherwise similar, conditional on observables, except for their tax preference—the magnitude of $e(t_i)$ increases. Among individuals in families with an employer-sponsored insurance policyholder who earns less than 50 or more than 150 percent of the maximum taxable wage, we estimate $e(t_i) = -1.28$. Other empirical studies that use very different methods report similar results. Gruber and Lettau (2004), for example, find an elasticity of firm-level insurance spending with respect to the tax price of −0.7; Smart and Stabile (2005) find tax-price elasticities of the demand for health services in the range of −0.7 to −1.0.

Based on these calculations, our estimate of $e(t_o)$ is 0.41 (= −.045 + 0.86). Thus, we conclude that making out-of-pocket spending deductible would lead to a decrease in health spending of 6.2 percent (= −0.15 × 0.41).

TAX CREDIT

The increase in spending attributable to the credit depends on what sort of insurance the credits' beneficiaries purchase. If they were to buy a policy that resembles that which currently insured individuals hold, then their spending would rise by 70 percent, from $2,290 to $3,885 per capita in 2008 dollars.[5] According to the RAND Health Insurance Experiment, a more modest insurance policy increases an uninsured person's health spending by 32 percent.[6] If we assume that the type of insurance obtained by people taking up the credit increases their spending by 50 percent, then the credit overall will increase health spending by $7 billion in 2010 (= 0.5 × $2,290 × 1.057 × 6,000,000).[7]

INSURANCE-MARKET AND MALPRACTICE REFORMS

The above estimates can also be used to calculate the impact of insurance-market and malpractice reforms on health care spending. In the text we reported that our insurance-market reforms and restrictions on "any-willing-provider" laws would reduce insurance costs by 7 percent. Because each 1 percent reduction in the after-tax price of insured expenditures increases total expenditures by 0.86 percent, a 7 percent decrease in the price of insured expenditures due to insurance reform would lead to a decline in total expenditures of about 1 percent (= 7 percent × (1 − 0.86)).

We also reported that malpractice reform would reduce the price of health care by 3 percent. Because each 1 percent reduction in the overall price of health care increases total expenditures by 0.45 percent, a 3 percent decrease due to malpractice reform would lead to a decline in total expenditures of 1.7 percent (= 3 percent × (1 − 0.45)).

TOTAL EFFECT

The combined impact of our policies is thus to reduce health care spending by 8.2 percent (= 6.2 − 0.7 + 1 + 1.7).

To translate this change into a dollar amount, we first transformed these percentage effects from arc-elasticity to point-elasticity terms. Arc elasticities represent the percentage change in spending relative to the average between the initial and final levels; point elasticities represent the percentage change in spending relative to the initial level. That is, if η is the percentage change in arc-elasticity terms, then η^* is the percentage change in point-elasticity terms, because:

$$\eta = \frac{\eta^*}{[1+(1+\eta^*)]\big/2}, \quad or$$

$$\eta^* = \frac{2\eta}{2-\eta}.$$

To determine how much each reform would reduce spending, we multiplied the η^* associated with it by the estimated 2010 level of health expenditures. According to CMS, private personal health care expenditures, excluding nursing home care, are projected to be $1,067 billion in 2010.[8] Thus, we project that our proposals will lower overall health care spending by approximately $84 billion (= $1,067 × 2 × 0.082 / (2 + 0.082)): $63 billion from deductibility, $10 billion from insurance-market reform, and $18 billion from malpractice reform less $7 billion for the credit.

The combined impact of our policies is not sensitive to our assumptions about the magnitude of $e(p)$, the responsiveness of health expenditures to their overall price. Even if $e(p)$ is half as great as we assume it is, the total effect of our package on health spending is 8.7 percent:

Tax deductibility: $e(t_i) = -0.43$, $e(t_o) = 0.2$, effect on spending $= 0.2 \times 0.15 = 3$ percent.

Tax Credit: $- 0.7$ percent.

Insurance reform: effect on spending $= 0.07 \times (1 - 0.43) = 4$ percent.

Malpractice reform: effect on spending $= 0.03 \times (1 - 0.2) = 2.4$ percent.

APPENDIX B

Estimating the Impact of Policy Reforms on Uninsurance

TAX DEDUCTIBILITY

To estimate effects of deductibility on the uninsured, we used estimates from Pauly and Herring of the elasticity of insurance take-up by the uninsured with respect to the price.[1] Pauly and Herring estimate that a 25 percent proportional credit would reduce the number of uninsured by between 13.3 and 38.9 percent. This reduction implies an elasticity of insurance take-up with respect to the price of between −0.53 (= 0.133 / 0.25) and −1.56 (= 0.389 / 0.25).

According to the National Institute for Health Care Management, approximately 20 million nonelderly uninsured individuals are in households earning at least 200 percent of poverty.[2] Assuming that each of these households has both a working member and pays taxes, we estimate that there are about 20 million uninsured who would benefit from tax deductibility.

The impact of tax deductibility on the cost of insurance for these 20 million persons depends upon whether their households have employer-provided insurance, which is currently tax-deductible, or whether they acquire insurance in the individual market, which by and large is not tax-deductible. For those in the individual market, the effect of the policy on the incentive to buy insurance is especially large because, by purchasing it, a person could deduct both insurance premiums and any out-of-pocket expenses, neither of which is deductible under current law. For example, consider a person who is contemplating the purchase of an insurance plan that costs $1,000 and would leave him with expected out-of-pocket expenses of $1,000. Assuming a marginal tax rate of 15 percent, this person would receive a tax reduction of $300, which translates into a 30 percent reduction in the cost of insurance. For a similar individual who has access to an (already tax-favored) employer-sponsored plan, the effect of the policy is still significant, but it is only 15 percent.

How many uninsured individuals are in each market? Pauly and Herring estimate approximately 60 percent of uninsured workers and their uninsured dependents—or 12 million persons—were not offered insurance by the workers' employers.[3] Hence, these persons are in the individual market.

Assuming a marginal tax rate of 15 percent and a catastrophic insurance policy that has out-of-pocket expenses equal to premiums, full deductibility leads to a reduction in the price of insurance of 30 percent. Thus, the reduction in the uninsured on account of deductibility lies between

2 million (= 12 × 0.30 × 0.53) and 6 million (= 12 × 0.30 × 1.56), depending on the elasticity of the take-up of insurance with respect to the price.

TAX CREDIT

The tax credit will further reduce the number of uninsured. Using the elasticities from Pauly and Herring and the population data in the text, we estimate that a 25 percent proportional credit given to individuals earning less than the poverty threshold (with a linear phase-out from 100 to 300 percent of the poverty threshold) will reduce the number of uninsured by between 3 million (= 46 × 0.21 × 0.25 credit × 0.53 + 46 × 0.47 × 0.25 credit × 0.53 × linear phase-out 0.5) and 8 million (= 46 × 0.21 × 0.25 credit × 1.56 + 46 × 0.47 × 0.25 credit × 1.56 × 0.5 linear phase-out) individuals.

INSURANCE-MARKET AND MALPRACTICE REFORMS

For insurance-market and malpractice reforms, we estimate that the total effect of exemption from state mandates and any-willing-provider laws and enhanced competition will be to reduce costs by approximately 7 percent; the effect of malpractice reforms will be to reduce costs by 3 percent. Given the range of elasticities of insurance take-up with respect to the price, we estimate that the insurance-market and malpractice reforms will reduce the number of uninsured by between 2 million (= 46 × 0.53 × (0.07 + 0.03)) and 7 million (= 46 × 1.56 × (0.07 + 0.03)) individuals.

APPENDIX C

Derivation of the Elasticity of Total Health Care Spending with Respect to the After-Tax Price of Out-of-Pocket Spending

We derive the relationship between the impact on health spending of making out-of-pocket expenses tax-deductible and two parameters from the economic literature: the price elasticity of health spending, and the elasticity of the coinsurance rate with respect to the tax preference for insured spending. We specify health spending E as a function of the after-tax price of health services relative to all other goods p and the tax preference for out-of-pocket spending relative to insured spending t_o / t_i, $E(p, t_o / t_i)$. In a world without taxes, p is the price of health services p^*. In a world with tax preferences, p is p^* multiplied by the weighted average of the tax preferences for out-of-pocket spending t_o and insured spending t_i, $p = p^* \times [ct_o + (1 - c) t_i]$, where t_o and t_i are weighted by the quantity shares of out-of-pocket and insured spending c and $(1 - c)$. The share c can also be thought of as the coinsurance rate, i.e., the share of spending out of pocket in the absence of tax preferences.

So

$$\frac{dE}{dt_o} = \frac{\partial E}{\partial p} \times \frac{\partial p}{\partial t_o} + \frac{\partial E}{\partial (t_o/t_i)} \times \frac{\partial (t_o/t_i)}{\partial t_o} = \frac{\partial E}{\partial p} \times \frac{\partial p}{\partial t_o} + \frac{\partial E}{\partial (t_o/t_i)} \times \frac{1}{t_i}$$

And

$$\frac{dE}{dt_i} = \frac{\partial E}{\partial p} \times \frac{\partial p}{\partial t_i} + \frac{\partial E}{\partial (t_o/t_i)} \times \frac{\partial (t_o/t_i)}{\partial t_i} = \frac{\partial E}{\partial p} \times \frac{\partial p}{\partial t_i} - \frac{\partial E}{\partial (t_o/t_i)} \times \frac{t_o}{t_i^2}.$$

Then the sum of these two equations, in elasticity terms, is:

$$\frac{dE/E}{dt_o/t_o} + \frac{dE/E}{dt_i/t_i} = \frac{\partial E/E}{\partial p/p} \times \frac{\partial p/p}{\partial t_o/t_o} + \frac{\partial E/E}{\partial (t_o/t_i)} \times \frac{t_o}{t_i} + \frac{\partial E/E}{\partial p/p} \times \frac{\partial p/p}{\partial t_i/t_i} - \frac{\partial E/E}{\partial (t_o/t_i)} \times \frac{t_o}{t_i},$$

or

$$\frac{dE/E}{dt_o/t_o} + \frac{dE/E}{dt_i/t_i} = \frac{\partial E/E}{\partial p/p} \times \left[\frac{\partial p/p}{\partial t_o/t_o} + \frac{\partial p/p}{\partial t_i/t_i} \right]$$

$$= \frac{\partial E/E}{\partial p/p} \times \frac{p^*}{p} \times \left[ct_o + t_o \frac{\partial c}{\partial t_o/t_o} - t_i \frac{\partial c}{\partial t_o/t_o} + (1-c)t_i + t_o \frac{\partial c}{\partial t_i/t_i} - t_i \frac{\partial c}{\partial t_i/t_i} \right]$$

$$= \frac{\partial E/E}{\partial p/p} \times \left[\frac{p^* \times [ct_o + (1-c)t_i]}{p} + [\frac{p^*}{p} \times (t_o - t_i) \times c \times (\frac{\partial c/c}{\partial t_o/t_o} + \frac{\partial c/c}{\partial t_i/t_i}) \right]$$

or

$$e(t_o) + e(t_i) = e(p) \times (1+\theta),$$

where $e(t_o)$ is the elasticity of spending with respect to the tax preference for out-of-pocket spending; $e(t_i)$ is the elasticity of spending with respect to the preference for insured spending; and $e(p)$ is the price elasticity of spending.

Simplifying this equation requires an estimate of θ. The first term in θ, p/p^*, is simply $[ct_o + (1-c)\,t_i] = 0.78$, assuming $c = 0.25$, $t_o = 1$, and $t_i = 0.7$. The second term $t_o - t_i = 0.3$, under the same assumptions as above. The third term $c = 0.25$. The magnitude of the fourth term is more difficult to assess, as it depends on the relative responsiveness of the coinsurance rate to the tax preference for insured versus out-of-pocket spending. As discussed in Appendix A, simulation models from the previous literature calibrate the elasticity of the coinsurance rate with respect to the tax preference for insured spending $e(c,t_i)$ to be around 1.9. Less work has been done to calibrate $e(c,t_o)$. However, based on the results in table 1 of Jack and Sheiner (1997), $e(c,t_o)$ is approximately -1. Thus, $\theta \approx 0.05$. In what follows, we assume $\theta = 0$ for simplicity. This leads us to underestimate $e(t_o)$—and thereby understate the impact on overall spending of extending deductibility to out-of-pocket spending—but only by a very small amount.

APPENDIX D

Estimating the Impact of Policy Reforms on the Federal Budget

Below, we provide details behind our calculations of the effect on the federal budget of tax deductibility, the tax credit, and insurance-market and malpractice reforms. All data are from the Centers for Medicare and Medicaid Services, National Health Expenditures Projections 2008–2018, unless noted otherwise.

TAX DEDUCTIBILITY

Gross revenue losses. To calculate the effect on the federal budget of tax deductibility, we first calculate the gross revenue losses from the policy. As described in the text, deriving gross revenue losses requires us to first calculate total non-deducted out-of-pocket spending and total non-deducted spending on health insurance. We calculate non-deducted out-of-pocket spending (OOP), net of spending on skilled nursing to be $166.4 billion:

Total OOP private personal health care expenditures
(excludes administrative costs), 2010
[CMS, Table 5] $292.1
   Less OOP spending currently deducted, 2010
   [see below]   −88.6
   Less OOP spending on SNF, 2010
   [CMS, Table 13]   <u>−37.1</u>
                         $166.4

Unfortunately, there is no similar comprehensive public
database available to identify the amount of after-tax contributions to health insurance by individuals. We calculate non-deducted spending on health insurance to be
$85.8 billion:

Nondeductible individual premiums, 2010 $52.9
[see below]
Non-excluded employee contributions to EHI, 2010
[see below]   <u>+32.9</u>
                         $85.8

We calculate currently deducted out-of-pocket spending to
be $88.6 billion:

Tax cost of medical expense deduction, 2010
[JCT, Table 1[1]] $12.4
   Divided by out-of-pocket spending-weighted
   implicit marginal tax rate   <u>/ 0.14</u>
                         $88.6

We calculate nondeductible individual premiums to be $52.9 billion:

Total household spending on private health insurance, 2007 [Table 6, Hartman et al. (2009)[2]]	$238.6
Plus 9.2% growth, 2007–10 (health services/ supplies) [CMS, Table 4]	+22.0
Less employee contribution to employer-sponsored insurance, private firms, 2009 [MEPS Table IV.A.1[3]]	−168.5
Plus 2.5% growth, 2009–10 (health services/ supplies) [CMS, Table 4]	−4.2
Less employee contribution to employer-sponsored insurance, state/local government health insurance, 2009 [MEPS Table IV. B.1[4]]	−27.6
Plus 2.5% growth, 2009–10 (health services/ supplies) [CMS, Table 4]	−0.7
Less employee contribution to employer-insurance, federal gov't, 2010 [see below]	−6.7
	$52.9

We calculate non-excluded employee contributions to employer-sponsored health insurance to be $32.9 billion:

Total private employee contribution to employer-sponsored insurance, private firms, 2009
[MEPS Table IV.A.1[5]] $168.5
   Plus 2.5% growth, 2009–10 (health services/
   supplies) [CMS, Table 4]   –4.2
Times the proportion of employee
contributions that are not excluded through
Section 125 plans
[Kaiser Family Foundation, Tables I and M.2[6]]   <u>× 0.19</u>
                                                                     $32.9

We calculate federal-government employee contributions to employer-sponsored health insurance to be $6.7 billion:

Federal government spending on private health
insurance, 2007
[Table 6, Hartman et al. (2009)[7]] $25.5
   Plus 9.2% growth, 2007–10 (health services/
   supplies) [CMS, Table 4]   <u>+2.3</u>
2010 federal gov't spending on private HI $27.8
Times the ratio of state/local government
employee contributions to health insurance
to state/local government employer contributions
to health insurance
[MEPS Table IV. B. 1]   <u>× 0.241</u>
                                                                      $6.7

Gross revenue gains. As discussed in the text, there are two components to gross revenue gains. To calculate the first, we first calculate the reduction in overall health spending, which we do in Appendix A. We multiply the reduction in over-all spending, $63 billion, by the health-spending-weighted average marginal income tax rate plus the health-spending-weighted average payroll tax rate, 0.32; this amount totals $20 billion.

To calculate the second amount, we estimate the increase in out-of-pocket spending, which we calculate as the difference between the reduction in overall spending and the reduction in employer-insured spending. To calculate the change in employer-insured spending, we first calculate the percentage change in employer-sponsored insured spending, relative to its initial level, to be

$$1-\left[\left(\frac{1-c'}{1-c}\right)\times(1+\eta^*)\right],$$

where c' is the coinsurance rate that obtains under full deductibility, c is the initial coinsurance rate, and η^* is the percentage change in point-elasticity terms in health spending from Appendix A. As in Appendix A, we use an initial coinsurance rate c of 0.25; we determine that the coinsurance rate that obtains under full deductibility c' is 0.333 because

$$c' = c\times\left[1+\frac{2(\eta/e(p))}{2-(\eta/e(p))}\right]\Big/ t_i,$$

where $2(\eta/e(p)) / [2 - (\eta/e(p))]$ is the implied rise in the after-tax coinsurance rate necessary to induce the spending decline in arc-elasticity terms; dividing by t_i, the after-tax price of health insurance (which we assume to be 0.7, as in appendices A and D), converts this to the rise in the coinsurance rate that must obtain.

To translate this value into a dollar amount, we multiplied the percentage change in employer-sponsored insured spending, relative to its initial level (calculated above) by total spending on employer-sponsored insurance (net of spending on skilled nursing), which we calculate to be $766 billion:

Total private health services/supplies (includes administrative costs), 2010 [CMS, Table 4]	$829.3
Less nondeductible individual premiums including skilled nursing facilities, 2010 [see above]	−52.9
Less private health insurance spending on skilled nursing facilities, 2010 [CMS, Table 13]	−10.4
	$766.0

Thus, we calculate the reduction in employer-sponsored insured spending to be $126 billion (= $766 billion × 0.164), which implies that the increase in out-of-pocket spending is $63 billion (= $126 billion − $63 billion). To determine the second component of the revenue gain—from the shift to out-of-pocket—we multiply $63 billion by the health-spending-weighted average payroll tax rate, 0.13; this amount totals $8 billion.

TAX CREDIT

We estimate the cost of the tax credit as the sum of two components—the cost of the credit for currently insured individuals plus the cost of the credit for newly insured individuals. To estimate the cost of the tax credit for currently insured individuals, we first calculated, using the 2002 Medical Expenditure Panel Survey, the cost of the credit, assuming its value would be $1,000 for individuals and $2,000 for families earning less than the poverty threshold, declining at a rate of 5 cents per dollar of income over poverty (approximately a linear phase-out over the 100–300 percent of poverty income range), and that all individuals with insurance would claim the larger of the deduction or the maximum credit to which they were entitled, given their family status. Under these assumptions, the estimated annual budgetary cost of the credit would be $20 billion. However, prior experience with a federal health-insurance credit and a considerable amount of academic research on health credits strongly suggest that the take-up rate for a new health credit would be less than 100 percent. In particular, the General Accounting Office's analysis of the 1991 health-insurance credit found that only 25 percent of the eligible population used the credit.[8] We have assumed a slightly higher take-up rate of 30 percent. Based on this estimate, we estimate the cost of the credit for currently insured individuals to be $7 billion.

To estimate the cost of the credit for newly insured individuals, we assumed that all 6 million recipients (the midpoint of the range of newly insured individuals due to the credit) were single and received the maximum credit of $1,000, which yields a revenue cost of $6 billion.

The net effect of the tax credit on federal revenue is the sum of these two components, or $13 billion.

INSURANCE-MARKET AND MALPRACTICE REFORMS

We estimate that insurance-market and malpractice reforms will reduce overall health spending by $28 billion (see Appendix A). Given that the new effective coinsurance rate, after full deductibility, will be 0.33, 0.67 of this transfer of health spending to other economic activities will be subject to both income and payroll taxation, and 0.33 will be subject to only payroll taxation. Thus, we calculate that the insurance-market and malpractice reforms will increase revenues by $7 billion ($= 0.67 \times 0.3 \times \$28$ billion $+ 0.33 \times 0.13 \times \$28$ billion).

Notes

CHAPTER 1. The Challenge: Obtaining High-Quality, Affordable Health Care

1. Paul Starr, *The Social Transformation of American Medicine* (New York: Basic Books, 1982).

2. Victor R. Fuchs and Harold Sox, "Physicians' Views of the Relative Importance of Thirty Medical Innovations," *Health Affairs* 20 (2001): 30–42.

3. See U.S. Council of Economic Advisers, Economic Report of the President (Washington, D.C.: U.S. Government Printing Office, 2002, 2004) for several recent indicators of American preeminence in health technology.

4. "Survey Results on Cost of Health Care and Health Insurance," Market Strategies, Inc.: Livonia, Mich. (2004).

5. The following statistics are from David Cutler and Ellen Meara, "Changes in the Age Distribution of Mortality over the Twentieth Century," in *Perspectives on the Economics of Aging*, ed. David A. Wise (Chicago: University of Chicago Press, 2004).

6. See David M. Cutler and Srikanth Kadiyala, "The Return to Biomedical Research: Treatment and Behavioral Effects," in *Measuring the Gains From Medical Research: An Economic Approach*, ed. Kevin M. Murphy and Robert H. Topel (Chicago: University of Chicago Press, 2003).

7. Mark McClellan and Daniel Kessler, eds., *A Global Analysis of Technological Change in Health Care: Heart Attack* (Ann Arbor: University of Michigan Press, 2002).

8. David M. Cutler, *Your Money or Your Life* (Oxford: Oxford University Press, 2004).

9. All figures are expressed in present value terms.

10. McClellan and Kessler, *Global Analysis*.

11. Richard Frank et al., "The Value of Mental Health Care at the System Level: The Case of Treating Depression," *Health Affairs* 18 (1999): 71–88.

12. OECD Health Data: 2010, available at http://www.oecd.org/document /16/0,3343,en_2649_34631_2085200_1_1_1_1,00.html.

13. Kaiser Family Foundation, *Employer Health Benefits: Annual Survey Summary of Findings* (Menlo Park, Calif.: Kaiser Family Foundation, 2000, 2009).

14. Gallup annual Health and Healthcare survey, conducted November 4–7, 2010, available at http://www.gallup.com/poll/144869/americans-ratings -own-healthcare-quality-remain-high.aspx and http://www.gallup.com/ poll/4708/healthcare-system.aspx, accessed January 22, 2011.

15. See, for example, J. P. Newhouse, "Medical Care Costs: How Much Welfare Loss?" *Journal of Economic Perspectives* 6 (Summer 1992): 3–21.

16. Mark McClellan et al., "Does More Intensive Treatment of Acute Myocardial Infarction in the Elderly Reduce Mortality?" *Journal of the American Medical Association* 272 (1994): 859–66.

17. Frank et al., "The Value of Mental Health Care at the System Level."

18. Martin Feldstein and Bernard Friedman, "Tax Subsidies, the Rational Demand for Insurance, and the Health Care Crisis," *Journal of Public Economics* 7 (1977): 155–78; Paul Ginsburg, "Altering the Tax Treatment of Employment-Based Health Plans," *Milbank Memorial Fund Quarterly* 59 (Spring 1981): 224–55; Amy K. Taylor and Gail R. Wilensky, "The Effect of Tax Policies on Expenditures for Private Health Insurance," in *Market Reforms in Health Insurance*, ed. Jack Meyer (Washington, D.C.: AEI Press, 1983); and Mark Pauly, "Taxation, Health Insurance, and Market Failure in the Medical Economy," *Journal of Economic Perspectives* 24 (1986): 629–75.

19. J. P. Newhouse and the Insurance Experiment Group, *Free for All? Lessons from the RAND Health Insurance Experiment* (Cambridge, Mass.: Harvard University Press, 1993).

20. U.S. Congress, Congressional Budget Office, *Increasing Small-Firm Health Insurance Coverage through Association Health Plans and Healthmarts* (Washington, D.C.: U.S. Government Printing Office, 2000).

21. Michael Vita, "Regulatory Restrictions on Selective Contracting: An Empirical Analysis of 'Any-Willing-Provider' Regulations," *Journal of Health Economics* 20 (2001): 955–66.

22. Daniel Kessler and Mark McClellan, "Malpractice Law and Health Care Reform: Optimal Liability Policy in an Era of Managed Care," *Journal of Public Economics* 84 (2002): 175–97.

23. Centers for Medicare and Medicaid Services, National Health Expenditure Projections 2008–2018, table 1.

24. Dahlia K. Remler, Jason E. Rachlin, and Sherry A. Glied, "What Other Programs Can Teach Us: Increasing Participation in Health Insurance Programs," *American Journal of Public Health,* 2003 93 (1): 67–74.

25. Jonathan Gruber, "Medicaid," in Robert Moffitt, ed., *Means Tested Transfer Programs in the United States* (Chicago: University of Chicago Press, 2003), 15–77.

26. Carmen DeNavas-Walt, Bernadette Proctor, and Jessica Smith, "Income, Poverty and Health Insurance Coverage in the United States," 2008, U.S. Census Bureau Publication P60-236(RV), September 2009, table 7.

27. See Robin Cohen and Michael Martinez, "Health Insurance Coverage: Early Release of Estimates from the National Health Interview Survey," 2008, Centers for Disease Control (June 2009) and May Chu and Jeffrey Rhoades, "The Uninsured in America 1996–2008: Estimates for the U.S. Civilian Noninstutionalized Population Under 65," Statistical Brief #259, Agency for Health Care Research and Quality (August 2009).

28. NIHCM Foundation Issue Brief, "Understanding the Uninsured: Tailoring Policy Solutions for Different Subpopulations," NIHCM Issue Brief, April 2008, table 1.

29. M. Kate Bundorf and Mark Pauly, "Is Health Insurance Affordable for the Uninsured?" *Journal of Health Economics* 25 (2006): 650–73.

30. See DeNavas-Walt et al. above.

31. NIHCM Foundation Issue Brief, figure 1.

32. Kaiser Family Foundation/Health Research and Educational Trust, "Survey of Employer Health Benefits," 2010, http://ehbs.kff.org/pdf/2010/8086.pdf.

33. Jack Hadley, John Holahan, Teresa Coughlin, and Dawn Miller, "Covering the Uninsured in 2008: Current Costs, Sources of Payment, and Incremental Costs," *Health Affairs* 27 (2008): w339–w415.

34. Helen Levy and David Meltzer, "The Impact of Health Insurance on Health," *Annual Review of Public Health* 29 (2008): 399–409.

35. See for example, the White House's discussion of the health reform law at http://www.whitehouse.gov/health care-meeting/proposal/whatsnew/affordability and the White House blog at http://www.whitehouse.gov/blog/2010/08/02/today-s-ruling-virginia.

36. Families USA, 2009, "Hidden Health Tax: Americans Pay a Premium"; Families USA, 2005, "Paying a Premium: The Added Cost of Care for

1111111

the Uninsured," Families USA Publication 05-101; and New America Foundation, 2006, "A Premium Price: The Hidden Costs All Californians Pay in Our Fragmented Health Care System."

37. See Daniel Kessler, "Cost Shifting in California Hospitals: What is the Effect on Private Payers," (draft) 2007, and John F. Cogan, R. Glenn Hubbard, and Daniel Kessler, "The Estimated Cost of Uncompensated Care for the Uninsured: Comparing Estimates from Three Studies," (draft) 2011, for an explanation of these flaws.

38. Jack Hadley, John Holahan, Teresa Coughlin, and Dawn Miller, "Covering the Uninsured in 2008: Current Costs, Sources of Payment, and Incremental Costs," *Health Affairs* 27 (2008): w399–w415.

39. Daniel Kessler, "Cost Shifting in California Hospitals: What is the Effect on Private Payers?" (draft) 2007.

40. For a comprehensive review of studies, see Sherry Glied, "Managed Care," in *Handbook of Health Economics,* ed. A. J. Culyer and J. P. Newhouse, volume 1A (Amsterdam: North-Holland, 2000).

41. "Survey Results on Cost of Health Care and Health Insurance," Market Strategies, Inc.

42. Robert Blendon et al., "Understanding the Managed Care Backlash," *Health Affairs* 17 (1998): 80–94.

43. Letter from Elmendorf, March 20, 2010, table 4.

44. John F. Cogan, R. Glenn Hubbard, and Daniel Kessler, "Obama's Gamble: Doubling Down on a Flawed Insurance Model," *The Economists' Voice,* Vol. 6 (2009), available at http://www.bepress.com/ev/vol6/iss10/art2/.

45. A recent *Health Affairs* article by staff from the Medicare Payment Assessment Commission suggests that traditional Medicare is beginning to suffer from exactly this problem. See Kevin J. Hayes, Julian Pettengill, and Jeffrey Stensland, "Getting the Price Right: Medicare Payment Rates for Cardiovascular Services," *Health Affairs* 26:1 (January/February 2007), 124–36.

46. As N. Gregory Mankiw has pointed out, this is precisely what happened with Fannie Mae and Freddie Mac: "The Pitfalls of the Public Option," *New York Times,* June 27, 2009.

47. Letter from Douglas Elmendorf, director of the Congressional Budget Office, to Nancy Pelosi, Speaker of the House of Representatives, on March 20, 2010. We arrive at the total of $935 billion by adding the following numbers from table 2: $465 billion spent on insurance exchanges and credits; $434 billion spent on Medicaid and CHIP coverage; and $37 billion spent on small employer tax credits.

48. Ibid. The first source of revenue, cuts to Medicare and Medicaid, totals $454 billion ($196 billion in cuts to the annual update to Medicare FFS

payment rates; $136 billion in cuts to Medicare Advantage; $36 billion in cuts to Medicare and Medicaid DSH payments; and $86 billion from "other Medicare, Medicaid, and CHIP savings"). The second source of revenue, new taxes, totals $452 billion ($32 billion in excise taxes on high-cost health plans; $210 billion in additional Medicare HI tax collections; $107 billion in taxes on health care goods and services; and $103 billion in other revenue provisions).

49. For example, according to the Kaiser Family Foundation Health Reform Subsidy Calculator (http://healthreform.kff.org/SubsidyCalculator.aspx), for a 55-year-old head of a family of four living in a high-cost area, the unsubsidized premium is projected to be $23,700 in 2014; the subsidy is projected to be $19,566. For the same family with an annual income of $95,000, the subsidy will be $0. For families in this income range, this translates into a total marginal tax rate of almost 100 percent—50 percentage points for the benefits phaseout, 15 percentage points for Medicare and Social Security taxes, 25 percentage points federal income taxes, and 5 to 10 points of state taxes.

50. For families in this income range, this translates into a total marginal tax rate of around 100 percent—50 percentage points for the benefits phaseout, 15 percentage points for Medicare and Social Security taxes, 28 percentage points federal income taxes, and 5 to 10 points of state taxes.

51. The employer mandate applies to full-time, full-year workers in firms that have 50 or more employees.

52. This incentive is intensified by the law's tax credits, available only to firms with 25 or fewer employees, to offset health insurance costs.

53. Katherine Baicker and Helen Levy, "Employer Health Insurance Mandates and the Risk of Unemployment," *Risk Management and Insurance Review* 11 (Spring 2008): 109–32.

CHAPTER 2. Five Policy Reforms to Make Markets Work

1. Melissa A. Thomasson, "The Importance of Group Coverage: How Tax Policy Shaped U.S. Health Insurance," *American Economic Review* 93 (2003): 1373–85.

2. Joel S. Newman, "The Medical Expense Deduction: A Preliminary Postmortem," *Southern California Law Review* 53 (1979): 787.

3. James W. Colliton, "The Medical Expense Deduction," *Wayne Law Review* 34 (1988): 1307.

4. DeNavas-Walt et al., "Income, Poverty, and Health Insurance Coverage in the United States: 2008," figure 7 (September 2009), 30.

5. Feldstein and Friedman, "Tax Subsidies," 171; and Charles E. Phelps, *Health Economics,* 2nd edition (Reading, Mass.: Addison-Wesley, 1997), 356.

6. Charles E. Phelps, "Large Scale Tax Reform: The Example of Employer-Paid Health Insurance Premiums," University of Rochester, Working Paper 35, 1986.

7. Authors' calculations.

8. E. B. Keeler, J. L. Buchanan, J. E. Rolph et al., "The Demand for Episodes of Treatment on the Health Insurance Experiment," Santa Monica, Calif.: The RAND Corporation, Report R-3454-HHS, March 1988. Amounts in text in 1984 dollars. In 2004 dollars (inflated using the CPI), the amounts are equivalent to an increase in deductibles from $364 to $909.

9. Ibid., table 5.3.

10. Newhouse, *Free for All.*

11. John F. Cogan, R. Glenn Hubbard, and Daniel P. Kessler, "The Effect of Tax Preferences on Health Spending," NBER Working Paper 13767.

12. Jonathan Gruber, "Taxes and Health Insurance," in James Poterba, ed., *Tax Policy and the Economy,* Volume 16, 2002, MIT Press, and the calculations in Cogan, Hubbard, and Kessler, cited above.

13. The Kaiser Family Foundation, *Employer Health Benefits,* reports that the average contribution was $6,656 in 2003.

14. U.S. Department of Labor, Bureau of Labor Statistics, "Health Spending Accounts," by Haneefa Saleem, *Compensation and Working Conditions Online,* 2003, http://www.bls.gov/opub/cwc/ cm20031022ar01p1.htm (accessed May 20, 2004). An employer may elect to allow individuals to carry over unspent Section 125 plan balances through March of the subsequent year. Internal Revenue Bulletin: 2005-23, "Modification of Application of Rule Prohibiting Deferred Compensation Under a Cafeteria Plan," June 6, 2005. http://www.irs.gov/irb/2005-23_IRB/ar11.html.

15. Julie A. Roin, "United They Stand, Divided They Fall: Public Choice Theory and the Tax Code," *Cornell Law Review* 74 (1988): 62.

16. U.S. Department of Labor, Bureau of Labor Statistics, "Health Spending Accounts."

17. Our calculations assume that the new tax deduction would apply to all medical and dental expenses that can currently be deducted under the IRS's minimum 7.5 percent rule.

18. 1977 is the earliest date for which Medicare cost-sharing data that are comparable to current data are available from the Centers for Medicare and Medicaid (see CMS, 2009, notes to table 4.1).

19. 2009 Statistical Supplement to the Health Care Financing Review, tables 3.2 and 4.1. The data are based on payments under Medicare's fee-for-service

plan only. Payments under Medicare Advantage and Prescription Drugs are excluded.

20. Copayments for inpatient hospital services, which tend to be less responsive to changes in coinsurance rates than physician services, have risen from 6.9 percent in 1977 to 9.4 percent in 2008.

21. See, for example, U.S. Government Accountability Office, "Medicare Physician Payments: Trends in Service Utilization, Spending, and Fees Prompt Consideration of Alternative Payment Approaches," GAO-06-1008T (2006).

22. The reduction in taxpayer-financed expenditures has two separate components. The first is the shift from taxpayer-financed expenditures to expenditures made by Medicare recipients as a result of the higher copayments. This reduction, 20 percent, occurs even in the absence of any reduction in the use of services in response to higher copayments. The second component consists of the reduction in program spending that occurs because of beneficiaries' behavioral response. As we discuss below, previous research on the privately insured non-elderly population indicates that the elasticity of health care spending with respect to the coinsurance rate is -0.45; that is, each 10 percent increase in the coinsurance rate generates a 4.5 percent reduction in health care spending. For a large change in the coinsurance rate, the appropriate measure of the percentage change is the total change, from 20 percent to 40 percent, divided by the average of the two coinsurance rates, 30 percent. This change yields an increase in the coinsurance rate of 67 percent and a corresponding reduction in total Medicare spending of 30 percent. Forty percent of this total accrues to Medicare recipients in reduced copayments, and the remaining 60 percent comes in the form of lower federal Medicare outlays. Thus, the total reduction in program payments equals $20 + 0.6*30$, or 38 percent.

23. Although it is possible that health spending in the elderly is less responsive to coinsurance than in the non-elderly, it is not necessarily so. One reason it may not be is that health care constitutes a larger share of senior citizens' household budgets than it does for younger families. Because income and substitution effects are additive, as the budget share of a good increases, its elasticity of demand increases, holding all else constant.

24. G. Shultz and J. Shoven, *Putting Our House in Order: A Guide to Social Security and Health Care Reform* (W. W. Norton & Company, 2008).

25. John F. Cogan, "Households Receiving Assistance from Federal Transfer Programs," (draft) 2009.

26. In addition, the 1996 Health Insurance Portability and Accountability Act provided protections to individuals' health care information and imposed additional rules, largely on employer-sponsored health plans.

27. Kosali Simon, "Adverse Selection in Health Insurance Markets: Evidence from State Small-group Health Insurance Reforms," *Journal of Public Economics* 89 (2005): 1865–77; Bradley Herring and Mark Pauly, "The Effect of Community Rating Restrictions on Premiums and Coverage in the Individual Health Insurance Market," NBER Working Paper 12504 (2006); and Anthonly Lo Sasso and Ithai Lurie, "Community Rating and the Market for Non-group Health Insurance," *Journal of Public Economics* 93 (2009): 264–79.

28. Susan S. Laudicina, Joan Gardner, and Natasha Stovall, State Legislative Health Care and Insurance Issues: 2002 Survey of Plans (Washington, D.C.: Blue Cross/Blue Shield Association, 2002); V. C. Bunce and J. P. Wieske, A State-by-State Breakdown of Health Insurance Mandates and Their Costs (Alexandria, Va.: Council for Affordable Health, 2010).

29. Bunce and Wieske, "Health Insurance Mandates."

30. U.S. Congress, Congressional Budget Office, *Increasing Small-Firm Health Insurance Coverage.*

31. Vita, "Regulatory Restrictions on Selective Contracting."

32. Frank Sloan and Christopher J. Conover, "Effects of State Reforms on Health Insurance Coverage of Adults," *Inquiry* 35 (1998): 280–93.

33. ERISA plans are not entirely free of federal restrictions on benefits. The Mental Health Parity and Addiction Equity Act of 2008, for example, requires that employers who offer a plan with mental health coverage provide mental health benefits "at the same level" as medical and surgical benefits.

34. Employee Benefit Research Institute, "Health Plan Differences: Fully-Insured vs. Self-Insured," Fast Facts #114, February 11, 2009, available at http://www.ebri.org/pdf/FFE114.11Feb09.Final.pdf, referenced September 20, 2010.

35. The following discussion is based on the excellent review in Hinda Chaikind, Bernadette Fernandez, Mark Newsom, and Chris Peterson, "Private Health Insurance Provisions in PPACA (P.L. 111-148)," Congressional Research Service R-40942 (April 15, 2010).

36. The community rating provisions require that premiums vary only based on age (by no more than a 3:1 ratio across age groups), tobacco use (by no more than a 1.5:1 ratio), self-only or family status, and geographic area (as determined by each state).

37. The law imposes the maximum out-of-pocket limits applicable to High-Deductible Health Plans on all individual and small-group plans (for 2010, $5,950 for single coverage and $11,900 for family coverage) and imposes maximum deductibles on small-group market plans of $2,000 for self-only coverage and $4,000 for family coverage.

38. Plans in the individual and small-group market, for example, are required to have minimum medical loss ratios of 80 percent. (The medical loss ratio

is defined as the portion of premiums that is spent on medical services as opposed to administration and profit.)

39. Minimum medical loss ratios (MLRs) both directly and indirectly discourage provisions that are designed to reduce wasteful medical spending. By definition, MLRs directly limit spending on administration, even if that spending controls health care costs and is in consumers' overall interest. In addition, because plans with greater cost-sharing necessarily spend a greater proportion of premiums on administrative expenses, MLRs indirectly discourage this approach to cost control as well.

40. John Cogan, R. Glenn Hubbard, and Daniel Kessler, 'The Effect of Massachusetts' Health Reform on Employer-sponsored Insurance Premiums," *Forum for Health Economics and Policy* 13 (2010).

41. H.R. 660, Small Business Health Fairness Act, 108th Congress, passed June 19, 2003.

42. L. Achman and D. Chollet, *Insuring the Uninsurable: An Overview of State High-Risk Health Insurance Pools* (New York: Commonwealth Fund, 2001).

43. Alan Monheit, "Persistence in Health Expenditures in the Short Run: Prevalence and Consequences," *Medical Care* 41 (2003): 53–64.

44. As noted in Marc Berk and Alan Monheit, "The Concentration of Health Care Expenditures, Revisited," *Health Affairs* 20 (2001): 9–18, these proportions have remained relatively stable from the 1970s to the present.

45. Joseph Newhouse, "Reimbursing Health Plans and Health Providers: Efficiency in Production Versus Selection," *Journal of Economic Literature* 34 (1996): 1236–63.

46. John F. Cogan, R. Glenn Hubbard, and Daniel P. Kessler, "The Effect of Medicare Coverage for the Disabled on the Market for Private Insurance," *Journal of Health Economics* 29 (2010): 418–25.

47. Stephen H. Long and M. Susan Marquis, "Potential Effects of HIPAA: A Review of the Literature," available at http://aspe.hhs.gov/health/reports/hipabase /pt2.htm, accessed September 20, 2010.

48. Bradley Herring and Mark Pauly (2006) have shown that regulation should not be necessary for guaranteed-renewable health insurance to be provided by the market under reasonable assumptions about the distribution of individuals' underlying health status.

49. See Carlos Zarabozo, Milestones in Medicare Managed Care, *Health Care Financing Review* 22 (Fall 2000) for an excellent review.

50. Kaiser Family Foundation, Medicare Fact Sheet/Medicare Advantage (September 2010), available at http://www.kff.org/medicare/upload/2052-14 .pdf accessed November 1, 2010.

51. KRC Research, "Seniors' Opinions About Medicare Rx: Fifth Year Update," September 2010, available at http://www.medicaretoday.org/pdfs/KRC%20

Medicare%20Today%20Survey%20of%20Seniors%20with%20Medicare %20Rx%202010%20FINAL.pdf, accessed November 1, 2010.

52. Statement by Paul Spitalnic, CMS Office of the Actuary, to *MedPage Today,* August 19, 2010, available at http://www.medpagetoday.com/tbprint .cfm?tbid=21761, accessed November 1, 2010.

53. Mark Duggan and Fiona Scott Morton, "The Effect of Medicare Part D on Pharmaceutical Prices and Utilization," *American Economic Review* 100 (March 2010), 590–607.

54. See Diane Rowland, "Medicaid at Forty," *Health Care Financing Review,* 27 (Winter 2005–2006): 63–77.

55. Julie Stone et al., "Medicaid and State Children's Health Insurance Program Provisions in PPACA," Congressional Research Service publication R41210 (April 28, 2010).

56. *Federal Register,* August 26, 2010 (Vol. 75, No. 165), pp 52530–52532, at http://frwebgate.access.gpo.gov/cgi-bin/getdoc.cgi?dbname=2010_register &docid=fr26au10-58.pdf.

57. M. D. Cabana, C. S. Rand, N. R. Powe et al., "Why Don't Physicians Follow Clinical Practice Guidelines? A Framework for Improvement," *Journal of the American Medical Association* 282 (1999): 1458–65; David Dranove, Daniel Kessler, Mark McClellan, and Mark Satterthwaite, "Is More Information Better? The Effects of Report Cards on Health Care Providers," *Journal of Political Economy* 111 (2003): 555–88.

58. Daniel Kessler and Mark McClellan, "Is Hospital Competition Socially Wasteful?" *Quarterly Journal of Economics* 115 (2000): 577–615. More recent work has found similar effects in the United Kingdom. See Zack Cooper et al., "Does Hospital Competition Save Lives? Evidence from the English NHS Patient Choice Reforms," LSE Health Working Paper 16/2010 (2010) and Martin Gaynor, Rodrigo Moreno-Serra, and Carol Propper, "Death by Market Power: Reform, Competition, and Patient Outcomes in the National Health Service," NBER Working Paper 16164 (2010).

59. Ibid.

60. Sean Nicholson, "Barriers to Entering Medical Specialties," National Bureau of Economic Research, Working Paper No. 9649, 2003.

61. See U.S. Department of Health and Human Services, "Addressing the New Health Care Crisis: Reforming the Medical Litigation System to Improve the Quality of Health Care," 2003, table 3.

62. Daniel Kessler, William Sage, and David Becker, "Impact of Malpractice Reforms on the Supply of Physician Services," *JAMA* 293 (2005): 2618–25; William E. Encinosa and Fred J. Hellinger, "Have State Caps on Malpractice Awards Increased the Supply of Physicians?" *Health Affairs* Web Exclusive, W5-250, 2005.

63. Kessler and McClellan, "Malpractice Law and Health Care Reform."
64. Susan O. Scheutzow, "State Medical Peer Review: High Cost But No Benefit—Is It Time for a Change?" *American Journal of Law and Medicine* 25 (1999): 7–60; Brian H. Liang, "Risks of Reporting Sentinel Events," *Health Affairs* 19, no. 5 (2000): 112–20.
65. Kessler and McClellan, "Malpractice Law and Health Care Reform."
66. Institute of Medicine, *To Err Is Human*.
67. For an excellent summary of these arguments, see Elizabeth Rolph, Erik Moller, and John E. Rolph, "Arbitration Agreements in Health Care: Myth and Reality," *Law and Contemporary Problems* 60, no. 1 (1997): 153–84.
68. U.S. Congress, Office of Technology Assessment, "Defensive Medicine and Medical Malpractice," OTA-H-602 (Washington, D.C.: U.S. Government Printing Office, 1994).
69. For a description, see ibid.
70. Gary J. Young and Kamal Desai, "Nonprofit Hospital Conversions and Community Benefits: New Evidence from Three States," *Health Affairs* 18 (1999): 146–55; Peter Cram et al., "Uncompensated Care Provided By For-profit, Not-for-profit, and Government-owned Hospitals," *BMC Health Services Research* 10 (2010): 90–103. See also Sean Nicholson et al., "Measuring Community Benefits Provided By For-profit and Nonprofit Hospitals," *Health Affairs* 19 (2000): 168–77, who find that nonprofit hospitals provide fewer community benefits than the level of investment in them would justify.
71. Mark Duggan, "Hospital Market Structure and the Behavior of Not-for-Profit Hospitals," *RAND Journal of Economics* 33 (2002): 433–46.
72. Kamal Desai, Carol V. Lukas, and Gary J. Young, "Public Hospitals: Privatization and Uncompensated Care," *Health Affairs* 19 (2000): 167–72.
73. Jack Needleman, "Nonprofit to For-Profit Conversions by Hospitals and Health Insurance," *Public Health Reports* 114 (1999): 108–1119; Young and Desai, "Nonprofit Hospital Conversions."
74. Daniel Kessler and Mark McClellan, "The Effects of Hospital Ownership on Medical Productivity," *RAND Journal of Economics* 22 (2002): 488–506.
75. William M. Gentry and John R. Penrod, "The Tax Benefits of Not-for-Profit Hospitals," in *The Changing Hospital Industry: Comparing Not-for-Profit and For-Profit Institutions*, ed. David M. Cutler (Chicago: University of Chicago Press, 2000).

CHAPTER 3. Impacts of Proposal on Health Care Spending, the Uninsured, the Federal Budget, and the Distribution of Tax Burdens

1. See, for example, William Jack and Louise Sheiner, "Welfare-Improving Health Expenditure Subsidies," *American Economic Review* 87 (1997): 206–21.
2. Congressional Budget Office, "Increasing Small-Firm Health Insurance Coverage."
3. Vita, "Regulatory Restrictions on Selective Contracting."
4. Matthew Eichner, Mark McClellan, and David Wise, "Insurance or Self-Insurance? Variation, Persistence, and Individual Health Accounts," in *Inquiries in the Economics of Aging,* ed. David A. Wise (Chicago: University of Chicago Press, 1998).
5. Ibid., table 1.1.
6. Monheit, "Persistence in Health Expenditures."
7. Ibid. The greater persistence of expenditures in this study is likely due to the inclusion of elderly and disabled people in the analysis.
8. For example, Christopher Hogan et al., "Medicare Beneficiaries' Cost of Care in the Last Year of Life," *Health Affairs* 20 (2001): 188–95.
9. Alan Garber, Tom MaCurdy, and Mark McClellan, "Diagnosis and Medicare Expenditures at the End of Life," in *Frontiers in the Economics of Aging,* ed. David A. Wise (Chicago: University of Chicago Press, 1998).
10. Mark Pauly, Allison Percy, and Bradley Herring, "Individual versus Job-Based Health Insurance: Weighing the Pros and Cons," *Health Affairs* 18, no. 6 (1999): 28–44.
11. This is the number of uninsured in 2008 according to the U.S. Census Bureau's publication P60-236, "Income, Poverty, and Health Insurance Coverage in the United States: 2008." To the extent that the number of uninsured people in 2010 is greater, our estimated reduction in the number of uninsured would be even larger.
12. Letter from Douglas Elmendorf, Director of the CBO, to Nancy Pelosi, March 20, 2010, table 4.
13. As Jonathan Gruber (2000) points out, empirical evidence supports the hypothesis that the costs of health insurance premiums are fully shifted out of wages.
14. Achman and Chollet, *Insuring the Uninsurable.*
15. See U.S. Bureau of the Census, "Health Insurance Coverage," table HI01. http://www.census.gov/hhes/www/cpstables/032009/health/h01_000.htm.
16. Based on authors' calculations using the MEPS Household Component Web tool, available at http:www.meps.ahrq.gov/mepsweb/data_stats/MEPSnetHC.jsp.

17. According to the Centers for Medicare and Medicaid Services, National Health Expenditure Projections 2008–2018, table 4, the estimated growth will be 14.5 percent.
18. Letter from Douglas Elmendorf, Director of the Congressional Budget Office, to Representative Nancy Pelosi, March 20, 2010, table 2.
19. http://budget.house.gov/pres_budgets/fy2011/hist.pdf, accessed November 30, 2010.

Conclusion

1. Milton Friedman, "The Drug War as a Socialist Enterprise," in Arnold S. Trebach and Kevin B. Zeese, eds., *Friedman and Szasz on Liberty and Drugs* (Washington, D.C.: The Drug Policy Foundation, 1992). See also Milton Friedman, keynote address presented at the Fifth International Conference on Drug Policy Reform, Capitol Hill in Washington D.C., November 16, 1991.

APPENDIX A. Estimating the Impact of Policy Reforms on Health Care Spending

1. For MEPS, Survey Instruments and Associated Documentation, see http://www.meps.ahcpr.gov/survey.htm, accessed July 7, 2005. For MCPI levels, see http://www.bls.gov/cpi/, accessed July 7, 2005.
2. W. G. Manning et al., "Health Insurance and the Demand for Medical Care: Evidence from a Randomized Experiment," *American Economic Review* 77 (1987): 251–77.
3. Matthew Eichner, "Demand for Medical Care: What People Pay Does Matter," *The American Economic Review* 88, no. 2 (1998): 117–21, table 1.
4. John F. Cogan, R. Glenn Hubbard, and Daniel P. Kessler, "The Effect of Tax Preferences on Health Spending," NBER Working Paper 13767.
5. Jack Hadley, John Holahan, Teresa Coughlin, and Dawn Miller, "Covering the Uninsured in 2008: Current Costs, Sources of Payment, and Incremental Costs," *Health Affairs* 27 (2008): w399–w415, Exhibit 5.
6. Emmett Keeler et al., The Demand for Episodes of Medical Treatment in the Health Insurance Experiment, RAND Report R-3454-HHS (1988), table 5.6.
7. According to Centers for Medicare and Medicaid Services, National Health Expenditure Projections 2008–2018, table 5, private personal health care expenditures are projected to grow by 5.7 percent from 2008–10.
8. Centers for Medicare and Medicaid Services, National Health Expenditure Projections 2008–2018, table 5.

APPENDIX B. Estimating the Impact of Policy Reforms on Uninsurance

1. Feldstein and Friedman, "Tax Subsidies"; Phelps, "Large Scale Tax Reform."
2. National Institute for Health Care Management, "Understanding the Uninsured: Tailoring Policy Solutions for Different Subpopulations," NIHCM Issue Brief, April 2008.
3. Phelps, *Health Economics.*

APPENDIX D. Estimating the Impact of Policy Reforms on the Federal Budget

1. JCT, "Tax Expenditures for Health Care" (2010), JCS-1-10.
2. Micah Hartman et al., "National Health Spending in 2007: Slower Drug Spending Contributes to Lowest Rate of Overall Growth Since 1998," *Health Affairs* 28 (2009): 246–61.
3. Medical Expenditure Panel Survey—Insurance Component, http://www .meps.ahrq.gov/survey_comp/Insurance.jsp.
4. Ibid.
5. Ibid.
6. Kaiser Family Foundation, Kaiser Survey of Employer Health Benefits (2007).
7. Micah Hartman et al., "National Health Spending in 2007: Slower Drug Spending Contributes to Lowest Rate of Overall Growth Since 1998," *Health Affairs* 28 (2009): 246–61.
8. U.S. Government Accountability Office, "Tax Administration: Health Insurance Tax Credit Participation Rate Was Low," GAO/GGD-94-99, April 1994.

About the Authors

John F. Cogan is the Leonard and Shirley Ely Senior Fellow at the Hoover Institution, Stanford University.

R. Glenn Hubbard is the Dean and Russell L. Carson Professor of Finance and Economics, Graduate School of Business, and a professor of economics at Columbia University. He is also a research associate at the National Bureau of Economic Research and a visiting scholar at the American Enterprise Institute.

Daniel P. Kessler is a professor in the law and business schools at Stanford University, a senior fellow at the Hoover Institution, and a research associate at the National Bureau of Economic Research.

WORKING GROUP ON
HEALTH CARE POLICY

The working group on health care policy aims to devise public policies that enable more Americans to get better value for their health care dollar and foster appropriate innovation that extends and improves life. Key principles that guide policy formation include the central role of individual choice and competitive markets in financing and delivering health services, individual responsibility for health behaviors and decisions, and appropriate guidelines for government intervention in health care markets.

The core membership of this working group includes Scott W. Atlas, John F. Cogan, R. Glenn Hubbard, Daniel P. Kessler, Mark V. Pauly, and Charles E. Phelps.

Index

tax(es) (*continued*)
  fairness and progressivity of, 44,
    94–95, 100
  increases to finance subsidies for
    uninsured population, 23
  marginal tax rates, 29, 35, 44, 89,
    100, 137n49
  PPACA on, 35, 38–39, 44. *See also*
    Internal Revenue Code; IRS
tax credits
  federal budget and, 90, 131–32
  health care spending and, 81
  in HSAs, 45
  impacts of, 7, 137n52
  for low-income households, 46–47,
    101
  McCain on, 38
  uninsured population and, 85, 119
tax deductibility, 2, 7
  under 7.5 percent rule, 44, 138n17
  after-tax price of out-of-pocket
    spending and, 80, 107–9
  of expenditures through cafeteria
    plans, 39
  federal budget and, 88–89, 125–30
  floor and ceiling for, 34–35
  full deductibility of health
    expenses, 40–44, 43b–44b
  health care spending and, 79–81,
    98–99, 107–13
  HSAs and, 7, 40, 45–46, 100–101
  of out-of-pocket expenditures,
    79–81
  percentage tax reduction and,
    93–95, 93f–94f
  uninsured population and, 43, 47,
    85, 99–100, 117–19. *See also* tax
    exclusion; tax preference
Tax Equity and Fiscal Responsibility
  Act (TEFRA), 63

tax exclusion
  for employer-provided insurance,
    27, 37–38
  for out-of-pocket expenditures, 34,
    39. *See also* tax preference
tax penalties, mandated insurance
  and, 25–26, 30, 137n51
tax policies, x, 2
  changes to, 100
  distributional impact of, 93–95,
    93f–94f. *See also* Internal
    Revenue Code; IRS
tax preference
  attempts to limit, 38
  Congress on, 38–39
  for employer-provided insurance,
    16, 27, 31–32, 34–38, 41–43,
    98, 110–12
  MEPS on, 36–37
  for nonprofits, 5, 74–75, 75b
  revoking, 35–36, 37, 98
tax reforms, 5
  markets, health care spending and,
    34–48
taxpayer-financed subsidies, 27–28, 29
TEFRA. *See* Tax Equity and Fiscal
  Responsibility Act
temporary "reinsurance" fund, 55, 60
Treasury Department, 39, 74
true insurance, 32, 41, 47

undocumented non-citizens, 21b
uninsured population
  causes and uncertain consequences
    of, 19–23
  CBO on, 21b, 87
  cost shift associated with treating,
    22–23
  effects of reforms on, 84–87,
    117–19

The Hoover Institution

The Hoover Institution on War, Revolution and Peace, Stanford University, is a public policy research center devoted to advanced study of politics, economics, and political economy—both domestic and foreign—as well as international affairs. With its world-renowned group of scholars and ongoing programs of policy-oriented research, the Hoover Institution puts its accumulated knowledge to work as a prominent contributor to the world marketplace of ideas defining a free society.

American Enterprise Institute
for Public Policy Research

The American Enterprise Institute sponsors original research on the world economy, U.S. foreign policy and international security, and domestic political and social issues. AEI is dedicated to preserving and strengthening the foundations of a free society—limited government, competitive private enterprise, vital cultural and political institutions, and vigilant defense—through rigorous inquiry, debate, and writing.